HEALTH CARE ISSUES, COSTS AND ACCESS

THE INDIAN HEALTH SERVICE

OVERVIEW, CONTRACT HEALTH SERVICES, AND AFFORDABLE CARE ACT IMPACTS

HEALTH CARE ISSUES, COSTS AND ACCESS

Additional books in this series can be found on Nova's website under the Series tab.

Additional e-books in this series can be found on Nova's website under the e-book tab.

HEALTH CARE ISSUES, COSTS AND ACCESS

THE INDIAN HEALTH SERVICE

OVERVIEW, CONTRACT HEALTH SERVICES, AND AFFORDABLE CARE ACT IMPACTS

PAMELA M. AGNELLI
EDITOR

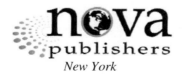

Copyright © 2014 by Nova Science Publishers, Inc.

All rights reserved. No part of this book may be reproduced, stored in a retrieval system or transmitted in any form or by any means: electronic, electrostatic, magnetic, tape, mechanical photocopying, recording or otherwise without the written permission of the Publisher.

For permission to use material from this book please contact us:
Telephone 631-231-7269; Fax 631-231-8175
Web Site: http://www.novapublishers.com

NOTICE TO THE READER

The Publisher has taken reasonable care in the preparation of this book, but makes no expressed or implied warranty of any kind and assumes no responsibility for any errors or omissions. No liability is assumed for incidental or consequential damages in connection with or arising out of information contained in this book. The Publisher shall not be liable for any special, consequential, or exemplary damages resulting, in whole or in part, from the readers' use of, or reliance upon, this material. Any parts of this book based on government reports are so indicated and copyright is claimed for those parts to the extent applicable to compilations of such works.

Independent verification should be sought for any data, advice or recommendations contained in this book. In addition, no responsibility is assumed by the publisher for any injury and/or damage to persons or property arising from any methods, products, instructions, ideas or otherwise contained in this publication.

This publication is designed to provide accurate and authoritative information with regard to the subject matter covered herein. It is sold with the clear understanding that the Publisher is not engaged in rendering legal or any other professional services. If legal or any other expert assistance is required, the services of a competent person should be sought. FROM A DECLARATION OF PARTICIPANTS JOINTLY ADOPTED BY A COMMITTEE OF THE AMERICAN BAR ASSOCIATION AND A COMMITTEE OF PUBLISHERS.

Additional color graphics may be available in the e-book version of this book.

Library of Congress Cataloging-in-Publication Data

ISBN: 978-1-63321-582-5

Published by Nova Science Publishers, Inc. † New York

CONTENTS

Preface		**vii**
Chapter 1	The Indian Health Service (IHS): An Overview *Elayne J. Heisler*	**1**
Chapter 2	Indian Health Service: Opportunities May Exist to Improve the Contract Health Services Program *United States Government Accountability Office*	**37**
Chapter 3	Indian Health Care: Impact of the Affordable Care Act (ACA) *Elayne J. Heisler*	**69**
Chapter 4	The Indian Health Care Improvement Act Reauthorization and Extension as Enacted by the ACA: Detailed Summary and Timeline *Elayne J. Heisler*	**93**
Index		**151**

PREFACE

This book provides an overview of the Indian Health Service. It also discusses the opportunities that may be available to help improve the contract health services program; the impact of the Affordable Care Act on IHS; and the Indian Health Care Improvement Act.

Chapter 1 – The Indian Health Service (IHS) within the Department of Health and Human Services (HHS) is the lead federal agency charged with improving the health of American Indians and Alaska Natives. It aims to do so by providing health services either directly or through contracts or compacts with Indian Tribes (ITs) and Tribal Organizations (TOs) to approximately 2.2 million American Indians or Alaska Natives who are members of 566 federally recognized tribes. IHS also provides grants to Urban Indian Organizations (UIOs) under the authority of Title V of the Indian Health Care Improvement Act. More than half of all federally recognized tribes operate facilities or health programs, and more than one-third of IHS's budget appropriation is administered by tribes.

The IHS health care delivery system serves federal reservations, Indian communities in Oklahoma and California, and Indian, Eskimo (Inuit and Yupik), and Aleut communities in Alaska. The system is organized into area offices, which are then further subdivided into service units. In FY2013, there were 12 area offices and 168 local service units. The IHS system is a mostly rural outpatient system focused on primary care. The system consists of five types of facilities: (1) hospitals, (2) health centers, (3) health stations, (4) Alaska village clinics, and (5) youth regional treatment centers. ITs and TOs may also operate other types of facilities or programs that exclusively focus on behavioral health concerns (such as alcohol and substance abuse). There are a total of 621 facilities in the IHS system; nearly half are health centers.

The IHS provides an array of medical services, including inpatient, ambulatory, emergency, dental, public health nursing, and preventive health care. The IHS does not have a defined medical benefit package that includes or excludes specific health services or health conditions. The majority of IHS facilities provide outpatient care, focusing on primary and preventive care including preventive screenings and health education. IHS provides services directly when possible; when needed services are not available, IHS beneficiaries may be referred to private providers for care. This is called purchased/referred care.

IHS also provides a number of health services that target common health conditions among IHS beneficiaries. These include services for diabetes prevention and treatment, behavioral health services including suicide prevention and methamphetamine treatment, and programs aimed at the prevention of infectious diseases. In addition to health services, IHS funds a number of activities related to its unique mission. These include construction and maintenance of IHS facilities, efforts to recruit and retain a skilled health workforce who will work at IHS facilities, and support for the overhead and expenses associated with contracts and compacts that the IHS enters into with ITs and TOs.

The federal government has long-standing involvement in Indian health. The Indian Health Care Improvement Act is the major authorizing legislation for the IHS. It was preceded by several laws that included more general authorization for federal Indian programs. A number of congressional committees exercise jurisdiction over legislation affecting the IHS, including its appropriations.

Chapter 2 – IHS provides health care to American Indians and Alaska Natives. When services are unavailable from IHS, IHS's CHS program may pay for care from external providers. GAO previously reported on challenges regarding the timeliness of CHS payments and the number of American Indians and Alaska Natives who may gain new health care coverage as a result of PPACA. PPACA mandated GAO to review the CHS program. This report examines (1) the length of time it takes external providers to receive payment from IHS after delivering CHS services; (2) the performance measures IHS has established for processing CHS provider payments; (3) the factors that affect the length of time it takes IHS to pay CHS providers; and (4) how new PPACA health care coverage options could affect the program. To conduct this work, GAO analyzed fiscal year 2011 CHS claims data, interviewed IHS officials, including officials in four IHS areas, and reviewed agency documents and statutes.

Chapter 3 – On March 23, 2010, President Obama signed into law a comprehensive health care reform bill, the Patient Protection and Affordable Care Act (ACA; P.L. 111-148). The law, among other things, reauthorizes the Indian Health Care Improvement Act (P.L. 94-437, IHCIA), which authorizes many programs and services provided by the Indian Health Service (IHS). In addition, it makes several changes that may affect American Indians and Alaska Natives enrolled in and receiving services from the Medicare, Medicaid, and State Children's Health Insurance Program (CHIP)—also called Social Security Act (SSA) health benefit programs. The ACA also includes changes to private health insurance that may affect American Indians and Alaska Natives and may affect tribes that offer private health insurance.

IHCIA authorizes many IHS programs and services, sets out the national policy for health services administered to Indians, and articulates the federal goal of ensuring the highest possible health status for Indians, including urban Indians. In addition, it authorizes direct collections from Medicare, Medicaid, and other third-party insurers. Prior to the ACA, IHCIA was last reauthorized in FY2000, although programs continued to receive appropriations in later years. The ACA reauthorizes IHCIA and extends authorizations of appropriations for IHCIA programs indefinitely. It amends a number of sections of IHCIA in general, to permit tribal organizations (TOs) and urban Indian organizations (UIOs) to apply for contract and grant programs for which they were not previously eligible; to create new mental health prevention and treatment programs; and to require demonstration projects to construct modular and mobile health facilities in order to expand health services available through IHS, Indian Tribes (ITs), and TOs. It also made several organizational changes to IHS. It requires IHS to establish an Office of Direct Service Tribes to serve tribes that receive their health care and other services directly from IHS as opposed to receiving services through IHS-funded facilities or programs operated by ITs or TOs. In addition, the law requires IHS to develop a plan to establish a new area office to serve tribes in Nevada and requires the Secretary of the Department of Health and Human Services (HHS) to appoint a new IHS Director of HIV/AIDS Prevention and Treatment.

In addition to reauthorizing IHCIA, the ACA includes a number of provisions that may affect American Indians and Alaska Natives who have private insurance coverage or who receive services through SSA health benefit programs. With regard to private insurance coverage, the ACA provides a special enrollment period for American Indians and Alaska Natives who may enroll in private insurance offered through an exchange and exempts certain

American Indians and Alaska Natives from the requirement to obtain insurance coverage. Under regulation, additional American Indians and Alaska Natives may also be exempt from the ACA requirement to obtain insurance coverage. With regard to SSA health benefit programs, the new law permits specified Indian entities to determine Medicaid and CHIP eligibility and extends the period during which IHS, IT, and TO services are reimbursed for all Medicare Part B services, indefinitely, beginning January 1, 2010. Prior to the ACA, authority for these facilities to receive Medicare Part B reimbursements for certain specified services had expired on January 1, 2010.

Chapter 4 – On March 23, 2010, President Obama signed into law a comprehensive health care reform bill, the Patient Protection and Affordable Care Act (ACA; P.L. 111-148). Among its provisions, the ACA reenacts, amends, and permanently reauthorizes the Indian Health Care Improvement Act (IHCIA). IHCIA authorizes many specific Indian Health Service (IHS) activities, sets out the national policy for health services administered to Indians, and sets health condition goals for the IHS service population to reduce "the prevalence and incidence of preventable illnesses among, and unnecessary and premature deaths of, Indians." The reauthorization of IHCIA in the ACA amends the IHCIA to, among other changes, expand programs that seek to augment the IHS health care workforce, increase the amount and type of services available at facilities funded by the IHS, and increase the number and type of programs that provide behavioral health and substance abuse treatment to American Indians and Alaska Natives.

This report provides a brief overview of IHCIA and summarizes the provisions of the Indian Health Care Improvement Reauthorization and Extension Act of 2009 as enacted and amended by Section 10221 of the ACA. Appendix A presents a timeline of the deadlines included in the act.

This report is primarily for reference purposes. The material in it is intended to provide context to help the reader better understand the intent of ACA's individual provisions at the time of enactment. The report does not track or discuss ongoing ACA-related regulatory and other implementation activities.

In: The Indian Health Service
Editor: Pamela M. Agnelli

ISBN: 978-1-63321-582-5
© 2014 Nova Science Publishers, Inc.

Chapter 1

THE INDIAN HEALTH SERVICE (IHS): AN OVERVIEW[*]

Elayne J. Heisler

SUMMARY

The Indian Health Service (IHS) within the Department of Health and Human Services (HHS) is the lead federal agency charged with improving the health of American Indians and Alaska Natives. It aims to do so by providing health services either directly or through contracts or compacts with Indian Tribes (ITs) and Tribal Organizations (TOs) to approximately 2.2 million American Indians or Alaska Natives who are members of 566 federally recognized tribes. IHS also provides grants to Urban Indian Organizations (UIOs) under the authority of Title V of the Indian Health Care Improvement Act. More than half of all federally recognized tribes operate facilities or health programs, and more than one-third of IHS's budget appropriation is administered by tribes.

The IHS health care delivery system serves federal reservations, Indian communities in Oklahoma and California, and Indian, Eskimo (Inuit and Yupik), and Aleut communities in Alaska. The system is organized into area offices, which are then further subdivided into service units. In FY2013, there were 12 area offices and 168 local service units. The IHS system is a mostly rural outpatient system focused on primary care. The system consists of five types of facilities: (1) hospitals, (2)

---

[*] This is an edited, reformatted and augmented version of a Congressional Research Service publication, No. R43330, dated December 3, 2013.

health centers, (3) health stations, (4) Alaska village clinics, and (5) youth regional treatment centers. ITs and TOs may also operate other types of facilities or programs that exclusively focus on behavioral health concerns (such as alcohol and substance abuse). There are a total of 621 facilities in the IHS system; nearly half are health centers.

The IHS provides an array of medical services, including inpatient, ambulatory, emergency, dental, public health nursing, and preventive health care. The IHS does not have a defined medical benefit package that includes or excludes specific health services or health conditions. The majority of IHS facilities provide outpatient care, focusing on primary and preventive care including preventive screenings and health education. IHS provides services directly when possible; when needed services are not available, IHS beneficiaries may be referred to private providers for care. This is called purchased/referred care.

IHS also provides a number of health services that target common health conditions among IHS beneficiaries. These include services for diabetes prevention and treatment, behavioral health services including suicide prevention and methamphetamine treatment, and programs aimed at the prevention of infectious diseases. In addition to health services, IHS funds a number of activities related to its unique mission. These include construction and maintenance of IHS facilities, efforts to recruit and retain a skilled health workforce who will work at IHS facilities, and support for the overhead and expenses associated with contracts and compacts that the IHS enters into with ITs and TOs.

The federal government has long-standing involvement in Indian health. The Indian Health Care Improvement Act is the major authorizing legislation for the IHS. It was preceded by several laws that included more general authorization for federal Indian programs. A number of congressional committees exercise jurisdiction over legislation affecting the IHS, including its appropriations.

INTRODUCTION

The Indian Health Service (IHS) within the Department of Health and Human Services (HHS) is the lead federal agency charged with improving the health of American Indians and Alaska Natives. The federal government considers its provision of these health services to be based on its trust responsibility for Indian tribes, a responsibility derived from federal statutes, treaties, court decisions, executive actions, and the Constitution (which assigns authority over Indian relations to Congress).[1] Congress is seen to have a moral obligation, not a legal one, to provide Indian health care.[2] Congress has reaffirmed its obligation to provide care to American Indians and Alaska

The Indian Health Service (IHS): An Overview

Natives in the reauthorization of Indian Health Care Improvement Act (IHCIA),[3] which is the major legislation authorizing most of IHS's activities. IHCIA stated that "it is the policy of the Nation, in fulfillment of its special trust responsibilities and legal obligations to Indians to ensure the highest possible health status for Indians and urban Indians and to provide all the resources necessary to effect that policy...."

IHS provides health services to approximately 2.2 million American Indians or Alaska Natives who are members of 566 federally recognized tribes.[4] The agency provides services directly or through contracts or compacts with Indian Tribes (ITs) or Tribal Organizations (TOs) under the authority of the Indian Self Determination and Education Assistance Act (ISDEAA).[5] IHS also provides grants to Urban Indian Organizations (UIOs), under the authority of IHCIA Title V, to operate health service programs. More than half of all federally recognized tribes operate facilities or health programs, and more than one-third of IHS's budget appropriation is administered by tribes.[6] In FY2013, IHS's appropriation was $4.1 billion.[7] IHS also receives a separate direct appropriation to support special diabetes programs[8] and supplements its appropriation with funds from collections for care provided to American Indians and Alaska Natives enrolled in insurance programs.[9]

IHS does not offer a standard set of medical benefits or services at all its facilities; rather available services vary by facility. These services are provided free to eligible American Indians and Alaska Natives (also called *IHS beneficiaries*) regardless of their ability to pay.[10] In general, IHS facilities provide health and health education services that focus on primary and preventive care. These services are available through a system of facilities operated by the IHS, an IT, a TO, or a UIO. These facilities are also referred to collectively as "I/T/U." (IHS/Tribal/Urban). They are referred to collectively as *IHS-funded facilities* in this report.

IHS services are available to members of ITs who reside on reservations and in non-reservation areas of those counties that overlap or abut reservations, and in some urban areas with a significant American Indian/Alaska Native population. Not all American Indians and Alaska Natives receive services from IHS, but more than half (58%) who are eligible do.[11] Those eligible for IHS may choose not to receive care at IHS-funded facilities because they are geographically inaccessible, because needed services are not available, or for other reasons.

This report provides an overview of the IHS and the population it serves. Specifically, the report describes the IHS's service population, the agency's organization, the type of facilities that IHS operates and funds, and some specific IHS programs that focus on reducing rates of common health conditions among IHS beneficiaries. The report also describes some other IHS supported activities such as those to construct new facilities, increase the IHS workforce, and support contracts with ITs and TOs entered into under ISDEAA authority. The report also describes IHS's authorizing legislation and the congressional committees that exercise jurisdiction over the agency. The report concludes with two appendices. **Appendix A** discusses how different federal agencies estimate the size of the American Indian and Alaska Native population. **Appendix B** is a timeline that provides a brief history of the federal government's provision of health services to American Indians and Alaska Natives.[12]

IHS USER POPULATION

The IHS user population differs from the self-identified American Indian and Alaska Native population because not all self-identified American Indians and Alaska Natives are eligible for or use IHS services. Specifically, IHS's user population was 1.6 million in FY2012;[13] in contrast, 5.2 million people self-identified as being American Indian/Alaska Native (either alone or in combination with another race) in the 2010 Census.[14] This section discusses IHS eligibility (including the broader service population) and how this differs from the self-identified American Indian and Alaska Native population. It also discusses IHS's actual user population and how this differs from the IHS eligible population. In addition, **Appendix A** includes information about how various federal agencies estimate the American Indian and Alaska Native population.

IHS Eligibility

Not all self-identified American Indians and Alaska Natives are eligible for IHS services; rather, to be eligible for IHS services, American Indians or Alaska Natives must be members of an Indian tribe (see text box for definition) or meet certain other requirements. In general, tribal membership is determined by the tribe. Many tribes require recognized descent from a particular tribal roll for membership. In tracing descent, tribes may follow paternal or maternal bloodlines, or both. Some tribes require minimum

The Indian Health Service (IHS): An Overview 5

percentages of genealogical descent, and others require only proof of descent. For a few tribes, Congress has set membership criteria in statute.[15]

In addition to tribal membership (i.e., meeting the IHS definition of Indian), certain other individuals are also eligible for IHS services because they:

- reside within an IHS health service delivery area, defined as a county where contract health services—also called purchased/referred care—are available;
- reside on tax-exempt land or have ownership of property on land for which the federal government has a trust responsibility;
- are recognized as an Indian by the community in which they live;
- actively participate in tribal affairs; or
- meet other relevant factors in keeping with general Bureau of Indian Affairs (BIA) practices in the jurisdiction for determining eligibility.[16]

A non-Indian woman pregnant with an eligible Indian's child would be eligible for care at an IHS-funded facility during the pregnancy and six weeks following birth, as long as paternity is acknowledged. The IHS also serves non-Indians in specific circumstances, such as emergencies or when an acute infectious disease is involved.[17]

IHS Definitions of "Indian" and "Indian Tribe"

IHS uses the definition in Section 4 of the Indian Health Care Improvement Act (IHCIA, 25 U.S.C. §1603) which defines "Indian(s)" as "any person who is a member of an Indian tribe." IHCIA defines the term "Indian tribe" to mean "... any Indian tribe, band, nation, or other organized group or community, including any Alaska Native village or group or regional or village corporation as defined in or established pursuant to the Alaska Native Claims Settlement Act (85 Stat. 688), which is recognized as eligible for the special programs and services provided by the United States to Indians because of their status as Indians."

Most IHS services are intended for members of federally recognized tribes, but UIOs may also provide services to members of terminated tribes— tribes whose federal recognition was withdrawn by statute—or to tribes that states recognize, but are not recognized by the federal government.[18] Members

6   Elayne J. Heisler

of terminated or state-recognized tribes are not eligible for services at facilities operated by the IHS, an IT, or a TO.

IHS User and Service Population

The *IHS user population* is a count of individuals who received care at an IHS-funded facility (including dental services and purchased/referred care services) one or more times in the prior three years.[19] IHS estimates that its FY2012 user population was 1.6 million.[20] This number is smaller than *the IHS service population* of 2.1 million, which represents the total number of American Indians and Alaska Natives who live within IHS service areas (i.e., American Indians and Alaska Natives who live on or near a reservation).[21] The service population is an estimate of IHS's potential user population (i.e., it includes individuals who do use IHS facilities as well as individuals who live near facilities and could use IHS, but have not done so in the prior three years). IHS estimates the service population using data from the decennial census conducted by the U.S. Census Bureau.[22] In non-census years, it adjusts the decennial census data for population changes using birth and death data from the National Center for Health Statistics, a center within HHS's Centers for Disease Control and Prevention.[23] Both the user and the service populations are generally smaller than the IHS eligible population because not all individuals eligible for IHS services live within the IHS service area.

IHS ORGANIZATION

The IHS health care delivery system serves federal reservations, Indian communities in Oklahoma and California, and Indian, Eskimo (Inuit and Yupik), and Aleut communities in Alaska. The system is organized into area offices, which are then further subdivided into service units. Service units may contain one or more facilities and may serve one or more tribes (see text box). In FY2013, there were 12 area offices[24] and 168 local service units.[25]

As shown in **Figure 1**, the 12 area offices generally cover one or more states with the exception of the Alaska area office, which organizes services exclusively in Alaska.[26] In contrast, the Nashville area office is responsible for IHS-funded facilities for states on the east coast, in Louisiana, and in parts of Texas.

The Indian Health Service (IHS): An Overview 7

IHS Service Unit
IHS service units are administrative entities within a defined geographical area through which services are directly or indirectly provided to eligible Indians. A service unit may cover a number of small reservations, or, conversely, some large reservations may be covered by several service units.

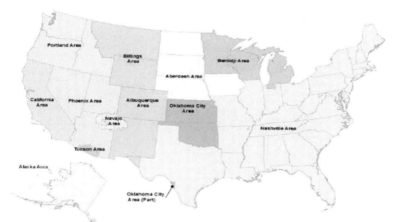

Source: CRS Analysis of IHS Provided Geographic Data.
Note: The figure does not include Hawaii because there are no federally recognized Indian Tribes or IHS-funded facilities in Hawaii.

Figure 1. Indian Health Service Areas.

IHS-funded health care is provided in facilities administered through area offices and service units. The 168 service units and specific health facilities may be managed either by the IHS directly, or by ITs, TOs, and consortia through self-determination contracts and self-governance compacts negotiated with the IHS under the authority of the ISDEAA.[27] ITs and TOs have taken over from IHS the responsibility for operating many service units and health facilities. More than half of all federally recognized tribes operate facilities or health programs and more than one third of IHS's total appropriation is administered by tribes.[28]

There are some geographic patterns in the location of tribally-operated programs, with certain areas having all or almost all facilities and programs operated by tribes. For example, the Alaska, California, and Nashville areas have few IHS-operated programs. Accordingly, these area offices are smaller because more funds have been provided to ITs or TOs to operate facilities and programs. In contrast, the Aberdeen and Billings areas have more facilities operated by the IHS.[29] In these areas there are relatively few tribally-operated programs, and area offices are larger than those in areas with more tribally-operated programs.[30] The size of the IHS user population also differs by area; more than one third of all IHS users live in two areas: Oklahoma City (Kansas, Oklahoma, and part of Texas) and Navajo (northwestern New Mexico, southeastern Utah, and northeastern Arizona, excluding the Hopi Reservation).[31]

IHS SYSTEM: FACILITY TYPES AND SERVICES AVAILABLE

The IHS system is a mostly rural outpatient system focused on primary care. The system consists primarily of five types of facilities: (1) hospitals, (2) health centers, (3) health stations, (4) Alaska village clinics, and (5) youth regional treatment centers. ITs and TOs may also operate other types of facilities or programs that exclusively focus on behavioral health concerns (such as alcohol and substance abuse). This section briefly describes these five types of facilities. As discussed above, the services available at UIOs differ from those generally available at facilities operated by the IHS, ITs, and TOs. UIOs and the services they provide are discussed separately below. (See report section "Urban Indian Health Programs.")

IHS Facilities

IHS, ITs, and TOs primarily operate five types of facilities. Of these, only hospitals and youth regional treatment centers provide in-patient care. The five types of facilities and the services they offer are:

1) *Hospitals (44 total)*: are generally small and services available vary by hospital. Some hospitals provide surgical services and specialty care services such as ophthalmology and orthopedics. Of the 44 hospitals operated by IHS or ITs, only one has an average daily census (a measure of usage) of more than 45 patients. Less than half of these 44 hospitals (19) have operating rooms.[32]

The Indian Health Service (IHS): An Overview 9

2) *Youth regional treatment centers (11 total)*: are inpatient facilities that provide substance abuse and mental health treatment services to American Indian and Alaska Native youth. Congress has authorized these treatment centers in each of the 12 areas (with California counted as two areas); however, two IHS areas— Bemidji and Billings—have opted to contract with outside providers for these services.[33] There are 11 facilities in total; five are operated by the IHS and the remaining 6 are operated by ITs or TOs.[34]

3) *Health centers (305 total):* generally provide outpatient services and provide primary and preventive care. Some health centers will provide health education and some laboratory, pharmacy, and radiology services. Health centers operated by ITs and TOs may also receive federal health center grants authorized under Section 330 of the Public Health Service Act.[35] ITs and TOs that receive these grants are required to provide certain services to non-IHS beneficiaries using non-IHS funds.[36] ITs and TOs may also operate school health centers that provide services similar to those provided in health centers to children during school hours.

4) *Health stations (108 total)*: are generally smaller than health centers; these facilities provide some of the same services that health centers provide such as primary care. One distinction from health centers is that these facilities are generally open less than 40 hours per week.[37]

5) *Alaska village clinics (164 total):* are unique to Alaska and may provide services using paraprofessionals assisted by health professionals via telehealth technologies. For example, Alaska village clinics operate the dental health assistant program whereby routine preventive dental care and certain less complicated dental procedures are performed by paraprofessionals at village clinics. These procedures are overseen by dentists who are available remotely.

Figure 2 shows the location of the five types of facilities noted above and depicts "other" facilities, which includes facilities or programs that address specific concerns like emergency care, or dental care (health centers may also include dental care). Within Figure 2, the locations of youth regional treatment facilities are within the broader category of behavioral health facilities.

Table 1. Number of Facilities Operated by IHS and Tribes (FY2013)

Type of Facility	Total	HIS Operated	Tribally Operated
Hospitals	44	28	16
Ambulatory (out-patient) facilities	577	97	480
Health centers	*296*	*61*	*235*
School health centers	*9*	*3*	*6*
Health stations	*108*	*33*	*75*
Alaska village clinics	*164*	*0*	*164*
Health facilities, total	621	125	496

Source: U.S. Dept. of Health and Human Services, Indian Health Service, *Fiscal Year 2014 Indian Health Service Justification of Estimates*, http://www.ihs.gov/BudgetFormulation/documents/FY2014 BudgetJustification.pdfcation p. 202.

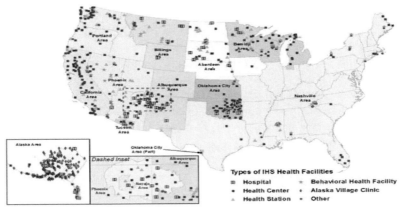

Source: CRS analysis of IHS provided data.

Note: The figure does not include Hawaii because there are no federally recognized Indian Tribes or IHS-funded facilities in Hawaii. The category "Other" includes facilities or programs that address specific concerns like emergency care, or dental care. Table 1 shows the total number of major IHS facilities by type of facility. It also illustrates that outpatient facilities are more likely to be administered by ITs or TOs than by IHS. The table does not include two of the categories included in Figure 2: "behavioral health facilities" and "other."

Figure 2. Locations of Indian Health Service Facilities, by Area.

Urban Indian Health Programs

Although most IHS facilities are located on or near reservations, IHS also funds, with approximately 1% of its budget, 33 urban Indian organizations (UIOs) that operate at 40 locations.[38] UIOs are supported by grants and contracts administered by IHS's Office of Urban Indian Health Programs. Services available at UIOs vary. IHS reports that 21 of the 33 UIO grantees provide direct medical care for 40 or more hours per week; however, the services available by facility differ. There are seven UIO grantees that provide direct medical care for less than 40 hours per week, with the number of hours ranging from 4 hours to 32 hours per week. There are also five grantees that operate outreach and referral sites that do not provide direct medical care, but provide behavioral health counseling, education services, and general health education services. Each of these five facilities has relationships with local (i.e., non-IHS funded) clinics to provide health care services to the American Indians and Alaska Natives they serve.[39]

UIOs provide care to approximately 51,000 American Indians and Alaska Natives who do not have access to facilities operated by the IHS, an IT, or a TO. In addition to IHS funds, UIOs may also receive funding from other sources, including state, private, and non-IHS federal grants and programs, reimbursements from federal programs, and from patient fees.[40]

AVAILABLE HEALTH SERVICES

IHS health services are provided directly by IHS-funded facilities (called direct services) or are provided indirectly under contracts with outside providers (called purchased/referred care services). This section provides an overview of services provided directly by IHS-funded facilities. This section also provides an overview of IHS's authority to collect reimbursements from federal health care programs and how these reimbursements are used to increase available health services. The section concludes with a discussion of services provided indirectly under contracts to IHS beneficiaries.

Direct Services Provided by IHS Facilities

The IHS provides an array of medical services, including inpatient, ambulatory, emergency, dental, public health nursing, and preventive health care.[41] The IHS does not have a defined medical benefit package that includes or excludes specific conditions or types of health care.[42] As noted above, the majority of IHS facilities provide outpatient care. The focus of services is on primary and preventive care including preventive screenings and health education.

Specialty services available through IHS-funded facilities are generally limited. Although some IHS hospitals do provide specialty care, services available vary by hospital. In addition, the IHS system, which covers a wide geographic area, only has 44 hospitals, which are generally small and provide limited services.[43] Some areas (e.g., California) do not have hospitals or may have only a few hospitals that may not be geographically accessible for the area's population (e.g., Bemidji and Nashville).[44] The absence or limited geographic availability of inpatient services means that some areas must contract with outside providers (using their purchased/referred care budget) to provide inpatient care and/or specialty care.

IHS also makes use of technology to expand services available at its facilities, which are often in remote areas serving small populations, thus making it difficult to provide specialty care efficiently. For example, IHS provides some behavioral health services via telehealth (e.g., counseling). Some facilities also use telehealth technologies to consult with specialists such as dermatologists or ophthalmologists when an on-site specialist is not available. The agency also uses these technologies to disseminate best practices developed in one IHS area to other IHS areas through training and technical assistance.

IHS also uses community members as paraprofessionals to provide care at rural and remote facilities. Specifically, IHS conducts a community health representative program, which provides training to community members who, in turn, provide preventive health services, health education, and follow-up care in rural and remote areas. IHS estimates that, in FY2012, ITs or TOs employed approximately 1,600 community health representatives.[45] IHS also uses dental health aides, another type of paraprofessional, in Alaska to provide routine dental services in remote Alaska Native villages.[46]

Collections

IHS facilities may supplement funding for services provided directly using reimbursements collected from Medicare, Medicaid, the State Children's Health Insurance Program (CHIP), the Department of Veterans Affairs (VA),

The Indian Health Service (IHS): An Overview 13

and from non-federal sources (e.g., private insurance).[47] IHS is unique among federal agencies in having this collection authority, and is able to retain these reimbursements to supplement the agency's annual appropriation.[48] IHS uses collections to augment funding available for clinical services. For example, reimbursements may be used to provide certain services (e.g., x-ray or other scans) that would have otherwise been purchased through the purchased/referred care program. Collections are retained by the service unit that collected them; therefore, service units have an incentive to increase collections because it enables them to expand services available at their facilities.

Health Services Purchased by IHS Facilities

IHS-funded facilities provide services directly when possible; however, when services are not available, IHS beneficiaries may be referred to private providers for care. This may occur in two ways: through the purchased/referred care (PRC) program or through the catastrophic health emergency fund (CHEF). Both programs are described below.

Purchased/Referred Care

IHS funded facilities may purchase care through contracts with private providers called purchased/referred care (PRC). These funds are limited because the program receives a discrete amount within IHS's annual appropriation.[49] The PRC eligibility criteria and requirements differ from those for direct services (i.e., services provided directly at an IHS-funded facility). The eligibility criteria differ in three specific ways:

1) To be eligible for PRC, IHS beneficiaries must live in specific geographic areas called "contract health service delivery areas" (CHSDAs).[50] CHSDAs are narrower than IHS service areas; therefore, it is possible to be eligible for HIS direct services, but not live in a CHSDA. CHSDAs are determined by each tribe, which could also mean that some tribal members may not live in the tribe's CHSDA, making them ineligible for PRC.

2) An IHS beneficiary may only receive authorization for PRC when the IHS beneficiary has exhausted all other health care resources available, such as private insurance, state health programs, and Medicaid.[51] This differs from direct services, where IHS can

encourage, but not require, a beneficiary to apply for alternate resources. For PRC, such applications and proof of denials are required.[52]

3) IHS uses a medical priority system to determine when a PRC referral will be authorized.[53] In general, PRC is only authorized for what is termed priority one services or "life or limb" services, meaning health services that are required to save a life or a limb.[54]

In addition to specific eligibility criteria, the PRC program has specific rules for patient and provider participants. For a patient to receive PRC services, an IHS beneficiary must be preapproved to receive the specific service. In case of emergencies, applicants must inform the PRC program within 72 hours.[55] For providers to participate in the PRC program, they must accept payment from IHS as full payment for services and may not bill an IHS beneficiary for authorized PRC services.[56] In the case of inpatient services, the hospital providing the service may only charge the PRC program what it would charge the Medicare program for the same service. This is called "Medicare Like Rates,"[57] but these rates do not apply to outpatient services; therefore, individual PRC programs must negotiate contracts with private providers to set rates for outpatient services.[58]

Catastrophic Health Emergency Fund

The catastrophic health emergency fund (CHEF) is a component of the purchased/ referred care budget that provides funding to reimburse costs for certain high cost cases (e.g., burn victims, motor vehicle incidents, high risk obstetrics, and cardiology). Unlike the PRC program that is managed locally and can be managed by ITs and TOs, the CHEF is centrally managed at IHS Headquarters. Local PRC programs can apply to the CHEF for high cost cases that meet the CHEF criteria. IHS has reported that there are more cases that meet the CHEF criteria than available funds.[59]

Disease or Condition-Focused Services

IHS provides a number of services directly or through ITs or TOs that target common health conditions among IHS beneficiaries. IHS also operates grant programs for ITs and TOs to target common conditions. The sections below discuss some of these programs. The discussion is not comprehensive; rather, it highlights some specific programs.

The Indian Health Service (IHS): An Overview

Special Diabetes Program

The Special Diabetes Program for Indians (SDPI) is part of IHS's ongoing National Diabetes Program administered within IHS's Division of Diabetes Treatment and Prevention program. IHS focuses on diabetes because the American Indian and Alaska Native population have the highest age-adjusted rates of diagnosed diabetes among U.S. racial and ethnic groups, a rate that is nearly twice the rate in the general population.[60] These high rates of diabetes increase health care costs for IHS beneficiaries. IHS's diabetes division, and the SDPI specifically, aim to reduce diabetes rates and rates of diabetes-related complications among IHS beneficiaries. With SDPI grant monies, the IHS, tribal ITs, TOs, and UIOs have set up diabetes programs to create an extensive support network that provides diabetes surveillance, health promotion, research translation, and other activities. As of January 2013, each area office had an area diabetes consultant and there were 19 model diabetes programs and 336 local community-directed diabetes program grants.[61] Since the SDPI's inception, performance measures have been used to evaluate the success of the SDPI efforts to fight diabetes. These measures have found increased blood sugar control, reduced cholesterol, and improved kidney function among IHS beneficiaries with diabetes.[62]

Behavioral Health Services

IHS beneficiaries have relatively high rates of substance abuse and mental health disorders compared to the general population; this is particularly true among younger IHS beneficiaries.[63] To address these issues, the agency operates special facilities to treat these conditions and administers a number of behavioral health programs, authorized in Title VII of IHCIA, through its Division of Behavioral Health.[64] In general, these programs aim to create a comprehensive behavioral health care program that emphasizes collaboration among alcohol and substance abuse, social services, and mental health programs. These programs also aim to integrate behavioral health care and primary care. Although some IHS-funded facilities have psychotherapy services for individuals and groups, in general, these services are not available 24 hours a day, nor are inpatient services available. Instead, PRC funds are used to provide after hours and inpatient services (except those services that can be provided at a youth regional treatment center). IHS-funded facilities also have programs that focus on suicide prevention, fetal alcohol spectrum disorder, and methamphetamine use because of high rates of these conditions among American Indian and Alaska Natives. For example, the

16   Elayne J. Heisler

methamphetamine and suicide prevention initiative supports 125 pilot projects focusing on innovative community-based interventions.[65]

Public Health Activities

IHS undertakes selected public health activities to encourage healthy behaviors and reduce the rates of infectious diseases. IHS does so, in part, because IHS funds are limited. Public health activities that prevent illness can reduce the need for certain health services, thus enabling the agency to expand its ability to provide care to its beneficiaries. Among other public health efforts, IHS employs public health nurses to prevent and undertake surveillance efforts of communicable diseases. IHS also devotes resources to increasing immunization rates, including a targeted effort to increase immunization against hepatitis B among Alaska Natives.[66] IHS also undertakes efforts to increase access to safe water supplies, thereby reducing the rates of certain diseases, through the sanitation facility construction program.

Prevention Activities

IHS prevention activities include funding for public health nurses who provide prevention-focused nursing care interventions for IHS beneficiaries and aim to improve health by screening and disease management efforts. For example, public health nurses work with IHS beneficiaries with chronic conditions to manage their care and reduce hospitalization. They also work with IHS beneficiaries who were recently discharged from a hospital to prevent complications and reduce rates of hospital readmissions. These services are provided in conjunction with health services provided at IHS health care facilities and focus on prevention to reduce the need for more intensive health care services. With IHS funds limited, prevention and screening efforts are an important component of the agency's strategy to maximize services available to its beneficiaries.

As part of IHS's prevention activities, IHS facilities make use of community health representatives (CHRs) who are community members trained as paraprofessionals to provide lay health education services, support patient self-management efforts, and improve health at the community level. CHRs provide health education, health promotion, and disease prevention services throughout the IHS service area. CHRs, like public health nurses, aim to prevent hospital readmissions and reduce emergency department use. They

The Indian Health Service (IHS): An Overview

provide a variety of services that include taking vital signs, providing foot care to diabetics, case management, and transportation services. They, like public health nurses, are part of IHS's efforts to expand the amount of services that the agency is able to provide.

IHS's prevention activities also include immunization efforts to reduce the rates of infectious of otherwise preventable diseases, including influenza, pneumonia, and human papillomavirus (HPV). In addition, IHS, with the Alaska Native Tribal Health Consortium,[67] undertakes efforts to increase rates of hepatitis B vaccination among Alaska Natives because the disease is more common in this population. IHS also undertakes vaccination and surveillance efforts to reduce disease rates and monitor and treat individuals who have already contracted the diseases.

Sanitation Facilities

Since 1960, under the authority of the Indian Sanitation Facilities Act,[68] IHS has funded the construction of water supply and sewage facilities and solid waste disposal systems, and has provided technical assistance for the operation and maintenance of such facilities. According to IHS in 2010, about 12% of American Indian/Alaska Native homes lacked safe drinking water supplies and adequate waste disposal facilities, compared to about 1% of all U.S. homes. IHS has found that this program has positive health benefits and is cost effective, providing a twentyfold benefit for every dollar spent.[69] Despite IHS's continued investment in sanitation facilities, there remains a backlog of approximately 3,300 sanitation facility construction projects. Fulfilling this backlog would require approximately $2.9 billion dollars.[70]

OTHER IHS-SUPPORTED ACTIVITIES

In addition to the activities discussed above, IHS funds a number of activities related to its role as a provider of health services. These include efforts to recruit and retain a skilled health workforce and to support the overhead and expenses associated with contracts and compacts that the IHS enters into with ITs and TOs to provide services.

Facility Construction and Maintenance[71]

The IHS funds the construction, equipping, and maintenance of hospitals, health centers, clinics, and other health care delivery facilities, both those operated by the IHS and those operated by ITs and TOs. ITs and TOs may handle these activities under self-determination contracts or self-governance compacts. The goal of these programs is to maintain IHS-funded facilities and the equipment within them. These funds are also used to ensure that IHS-funded facilities meet applicable building codes and standards, including those needed in order to be accredited by the relevant health care accreditation body for the facility type (e.g., The Joint Commission provides accreditation for hospitals).[72] Such accreditation may be needed to receive reimbursements from Medicare, Medicaid, CHIP, the VA, and private insurance plans. IHS also funds the construction of new facilities using a priority system that IHS developed with ITs and TOs to determine the order in which new facilities are built.

Indian Health Workforce

IHS, like other types of health care facilities located in rural areas, often has health care provider vacancies because of difficulty attracting and retaining health care professionals.[73] For example, the agency's vacancy rate in 2013 was 20% for physicians and 15% for nurses.[74] As one mechanism to fill these vacancies, IHS administers programs to recruit and retain providers including a scholarship program and a loan repayment program. The IHS scholarship program targets American Indians and Alaska Natives who are training in the health professions and provides academic support (including stipends) in exchange for a commitment to provide care, for a specified period of time, at an IHS-funded facility at the completion of their training.[75] Similarly, IHS provides loan repayments to health professionals (who may or may not be American Indian or Alaska Native) in exchange for a service commitment at an IHS-funded facility.[76] In addition to these programs, IHS also provides recruitment bonuses and bonus pay to make IHS salaries for health providers more competitive with the private sector. These programs are generally used to recruit for health professions with the highest vacancy rates or for health facilities that have difficultly recruiting providers (e.g., because they are in remote locations).[77]

IHS also partners with the Health Resources and Services Administration (HRSA), the HHS agency that is the lead federal agency on health workforce policy, to obtain providers from the National Health Service Corps (NHSC). The NHSC is HRSA's scholarship and loan repayment program where providers receive support in exchange for a commitment to provide care in a health professions shortage area, including at an IHS-funded facility. As of February 2013, IHS reports that there were 588 IHS health facilities designated as having provider shortages, and therefore eligible to receive NHSC providers, and 305 NHSC providers were located at IHS facilities. IHS reports that this collaboration enabled the agency to provide an additional 188,500 patient visits.[78]

Contract Support Costs

IHS, through its annual appropriation, provides contract support costs (CSCs) to ITs and TOs to help pay the costs of administering IHS-funded programs under self-determination contracts or self-governance compacts authorized by ISDEAA.[79] CSC pays for costs that tribes incur for such items as financial management, accounting, training, and program start-up. ITs and TOs have often complained about CSC funding shortfalls and note that these shortfalls have resulted in reduced services or decreased administrative efficiency for tribes with contracts and compacts.[80] A 2012 Supreme Court decision—*Salazar v. Ramah Navajo*[81]—required that IHS have sufficient CSCs available to support the contracts it enters into. Specifically, the Court held that a lack of appropriations did not release the federal government from its obligations to fully reimburse CSC costs. As a result of the decision, IHS is balancing the competing priorities of ITs' and TOs' desires to administer their own programs with the amount of CSC funds available. IHS says it must ensure that adequate CSC funds are available for existing contracts and that new contracts the agency enters into do not offset funding available for direct health care services.[82]

IHS AUTHORIZATION

The Indian Health Care Improvement Act (IHCIA, P.L. 94-437, as amended) is the major authorizing legislation for the IHS. It was preceded by several laws that included more general authorization for federal Indian

20 Elayne J. Heisler

programs. This section briefly describes several of these laws beginning from oldest to the most recent. See also **Appendix B** for a timeline of when these laws were enacted.

Snyder Act of 1921[83]

In 1921, Congress enacted the Snyder Act, which provided broad and permanent authorization for federal Indian programs, including health-related programs. The law provided the BIA, within the Department of the Interior, explicit authorization for much of the activities that the agency was already undertaking. It also authorized the employment of physicians to serve Indian tribes. Prior to the Snyder Act, Congress had made detailed annual appropriations for these BIA activities, but funds were not always appropriated because these activities lacked an explicit authorization. The Snyder Act provided an explicit authorization for nearly any Indian program, including health care, for which Congress enacts appropriations. The Snyder Act did not require any specific programs.

Indian Health Facilities Act (Transfer Act) of 1954[84]

In 1954, Congress enacted the Transfer Act of 1954, which transferred the responsibility for Indian health care from the BIA to the Public Health Service (PHS) in the then newly established Department of Health, Education and Welfare (now HHS). This transfer occurred because, among other reasons, Congress felt that the PHS could do a better job of providing health care services to Indians.[85]

Indian Sanitation Facilities Act of 1959[86]

In 1959, Congress enacted the Indian Sanitation Facility Act, which amended the Transfer Act and authorized the PHS to construct sanitation facilities for Indian communities and homes. IHS estimates that the construction of sanitation facilities has reduced rates of infant mortality, mortality from gastroenteritis and environmentally related diseases by 80% since 1973.[87]

Indian Self-Determination and Education Assistance Act (ISDEAA) of 1975[88]

In 1975, Congress enacted ISDEAA, which provided for the tribal administration of federal Indian programs, especially BIA and IHS programs. The act permits tribes to assume some control over the management of their health care services by negotiating "self-determination contracts" with IHS for tribal management of specific IHS programs. Under a self-determination contract, IHS transfers to tribal control the funds it would have spent for the contracted program so the tribe might operate the program. Under ISDEAA authority, IHS has also established a tribal consultation policy giving tribes an opportunity to help formulate health priorities in the President's annual budget request.

Indian Health Care Improvement Act (IHCIA) of 1976[89]

In 1976, Congress enacted IHCIA, which authorized many specific IHS activities, sets out the national policy for health services administered to Indians, and set health condition goals for the IHS service population. Most significantly, IHCIA authorized collections from Medicare, Medicaid, and other third party insurers and established a demonstration project for ITs and TOs to directly receive reimbursements. It also gave IHS authority to grant funding to UIOs to provide health care services to urban Indians and established substance abuse treatment programs, and Indian health professions recruitment programs, among others. The IHCIA was reauthorized by the Indian Health Amendments of 1992,[90] which extended authorizations of its appropriations through FY2000. The authorizations for all IHCIA programs were later extended through FY2001.[91] Although IHCIA-authorized programs continued to receive appropriations, the IHCIA was not again reauthorized until the Patient Protection and Affordable Care Act (ACA) was enacted on March 23, 2010.[92] The ACA reauthorized IHCIA permanently and indefinitely (see "Patient Protection and Affordable Care Act of 2010").

Indian Health Amendments of 1992[93]

In 1992, Congress enacted the Indian Health Amendments of 1992, which reauthorized IHCIA and amended ISDEAA to permit tribal governments to consolidate IHS self-determination contracts for multiple IHS programs into a single "self-governance compact." Self-governance compacts are similar to self-determination contracts as IHS transfers funds and operating control to a tribe, but the compacting tribe is then authorized to redesign programs and services and to reallocate funds for those programs and services. The 1992 amendment paralleled a 1988 change whereby the BIA allowed, under a demonstration, its programs to be compacted.[94] In 2000, the Tribal Self-Governance Amendments[95] made the IHS self-governance program permanent by further amending ISDEAA to create Title V, which included an authorization for self-governance compacts.

Alaska Native and American Indian Direct Reimbursement Act of 2000[96]

In 2000, Congress enacted the Alaska Native and American Indian Direct Reimbursement Act that made permanent the IHCIA demonstration program that allowed facilities operated by ITs and TOs to directly bill Medicare, Medicaid, and other third-party payors. The demonstration program, involving four tribally operated IHS-owned hospitals and clinics, had increased collections, reduced the turn-around time between billing and receipt of payment, eased tracking of billings and collections, and reduced administrative costs.

Patient Protection and Affordable Care Act of 2010[97]

In 2010, Congress enacted the ACA, which among other things, permanently reauthorized the IHCIA. The reauthorization expanded IHS activities to include long-term care services, created a continuum of behavioral health and treatment services, and expanded the ability of ITs and TOs to receive reimbursements directly from Medicare and Medicaid.[98] The ACA also included other changes that may affect IHS, such as expansions of access to private insurance coverage that may result in more IHS beneficiaries having private insurance coverage, expanded reimbursements for certain Medicare services provided at IHS-funded facilities, and changes in the way private insurance plans offered by ITs and TOS are treated for tax purposes.[99]

The Indian Health Service (IHS): An Overview

Table 2. IHS Committee Jurisdiction

House	Senate
Natural Resources: Holds jurisdiction for Indian health care and self-governance related legislation. **Energy and Commerce-** Holds jurisdiction for matters related to public health, Medicaid, the State Children's Health Insurance Program (CHIP), and shares jurisdiction for Medicare Part B with Ways and Means. **Ways and Means-** Shares jurisdiction for Medicare Part B with Energy and Commerce and has jurisdiction for Medicare Part A. **Appropriations (subcommittee on Interior and Environment and Related Agencies):** Holds jurisdiction for IHS appropriations. This differs from the appropriations of most HHS (and PHS agencies) that are under the jurisdiction of the subcommittee on Labor, Health and Human Services, Education, and Related Agencies.	**Committee on Indian Affairs:** Holds jurisdiction over all issues related to Indians. **Health, Education, Labor, and Pensions:** Holds jurisdiction over matters related to public health. **Finance:** Holds jurisdiction over Medicare (all parts), Medicaid, and CHIP. **Appropriations (subcommittee on Interior and Environment and Related Agencies):** Holds jurisdiction for IHS appropriations. This differs from the appropriations of most HHS (and PHS agencies) that are under the jurisdiction of the subcommittee on Labor, Health and Human Services, Education, and Related Agencies.

Source: CRS Analysis of congressional Committee structure. For information on which services are included in Medicare Parts and A and B, see CRS Report R40425, *Medicare Primer*, coordinated by Patricia A. Davis and Scott R. Talaga.

CONGRESSIONAL COMMITTEE JURISDICTION

A number of congressional committees exercise jurisdiction over legislation affecting the IHS, including its appropriations. These various committees are described in **Table 2** above.

24   Elayne J. Heisler

In general, legislation amending an existing statute is likely to be referred to the committees that exercised jurisdiction over the original legislation. IHCIA included authorization for participation in Medicare, Medicaid, and CHIP. As such, the committees that have oversight over these programs have been involved in the IHCIA reauthorization. In addition, these committees have oversight over legislation that affects IHS beneficiary participation in these programs and the ability of IHS-funded facilities to receive reimbursements from these programs.

CONCLUSION

IHS provides health care to American Indians and Alaska Natives who live on or near Indian reservations or in Alaska Native villages. Although IHS services are available free of charge to all eligible beneficiaries, not all eligible individuals choose to receive care at an IHS-funded facility.

This may occur because facilities are geographically inconvenient or because needed services are unavailable. IHS focuses on primary and preventive services, so some services may not be available. Despite this, IHS has attempted to expand services by partnering with local providers, by using technology and paraprofessionals to expand the services that the agency can provide at its facilities, and by preventing disease and encouraging healthy behaviors to reduce the need for expensive health services.

APPENDIX A. THE AMERICAN INDIAN AND ALASKA NATIVE POPULATION

There is no uniform definition of the American Indian and Alaska Native population. Rather, federal agencies use different definitions of this population. The Indian Health Service (IHS) service population data are based on U.S. Census Bureau data, which use self-identification as American Indian/Alaska Native by race, not tribal membership.[100] Beginning with the 2000 Census,[101] respondents were permitted to identify as members of more than one race or ethnic group.

Consequently, some individuals who might have previously self-identified as another race, beginning in 2000, were allowed to also identify as American Indian or Alaska Natives. As such, the number of American Indians and

The Indian Health Service (IHS): An Overview

Alaska Natives identified increased between the 1990 and 2000 Censuses beyond what would have been expected due to population growth alone.

The population also increased between 2000 and 2010 Censuses. Census 2010 found that 3.7 million people identified themselves as being American Indian/Alaska Native alone and 1.5 million identified as being American Indian/Alaska Native and another race, for a total of 5.2 million people, or a 21% increase from Census 2000.[102]

Tribes vary on their definitions of membership; some tribes may reserve membership for those whose parents were both members, while other tribes may trace membership to a grandparent or parent who is a member. Thus, in some cases, tribal members could be counted by the Census as American Indian or Alaska Native and a member of another race. Conversely, some individuals identifying as multiple races in the Census may not be tribal members. Given this and the fact that not all tribes are federally recognized, not all American Indian/Alaska Natives (either alone or in combination with another race) counted by the Census are eligible for IHS services. Despite the limitations of the Census data, IHS uses Census data to estimate its eligible population. In addition to imprecise estimates of the eligible population, IHS also estimates its "user population," based on registered American Indian/Alaska Native patients who used IHS-funded services at least once in the most recent three years.[103] This figure, estimated at 2.1 million in 2012, is lower than the eligible population because not all eligible American Indian/Alaska Natives received IHS services during the reference period.[104]

The Bureau of Indian Affairs (BIA) within the Department of the Interior also collects data on its service population, but uses a different definition than both IHS and the Census Bureau. BIA data are based on estimates received from BIA agencies and federally recognized tribes, but these estimates are not based on actual censuses and cover only persons on or near reservations.[105] The BIA also lists tribes' reports of their enrollment totals, but the BIA conducts no census to confirm these figures, and its publication does not show whether the enrollees enumerated live on or near reservations or inside or outside IHS service areas. In addition to these limitations, available BIA data are dated because the agency has not published data since 2005. **Table A-1** compares recent IHS, BIA, and Census population figures.

Determining the *urban* Indian population eligible for Urban Indian Health Program services is equally inexact. Urban Indian Organizations (UIOs) serve a wider range of eligible persons, including members of terminated or state-recognized tribes and their children and grandchildren (see report section "Urban Indian Health Programs"). They are not, however, authorized to serve

26   Elayne J. Heisler

anyone who merely identifies themselves as racially American Indian or Alaska Native.[106]

BIA figures for service population and tribal enrollment do not help determine the urban UIO population, because the BIA data are not broken down by urban or metropolitan residence, nor do they cover terminated or state-recognized tribes.

Nor is an answer provided by Census Bureau data on American Indians/Alaska Natives, since, although the data are broken down by urban, metropolitan, city, and other types of residence, they are still, as noted above, based on self-identification by race, not on tribal membership, whether in federal, state, or terminated tribes. IHS figures for urban Indian populations are based on these Census data.

Table A-1. Differing Indian Population Figures, Selected Years, 1990-2012

Year	Indian Health Service (IHS)		Bureau of Indian Affairs (BIA)[a]		Census Bureau	
	Service Population (in IHS service areas; est.)	User Population (at IHS facilities)	Service Population (on or near reservations; est.)[b]	Tribal Enrollment (national; est.)	American Indian/Alaska Native race alone (est.)[c]	American Indian/Alaska Native Race Alone or in Combination with Other Races (est.)[d]
1990	1,207,236	1,104,693	—	—	Decennial: 1,959,234	—
1991	1,242,745	1,134,655	1,001,606	—	2,187,000	—
1997	1,427,453	1,300,634	1,442,747	1,654,433	2,290,000	—
1999	1,489,341	—	1,397,931	1,698,483	2,397,000	—
2000	1,641,828	—	—	—	Decennial: 2,475,956	Decennial: 4,119,301
2001	1,670,454	1,345,242	1,524,025	1,816,504	2,725,594	4,319,387
2003	1,744,792	1,383,664	1,587,519	1,923,650	2,821,438	4,464,402
2005	1,805,122	—	1,731,178	1,978,099	2,924,141	4,620,280
2006	1,829,792	1,461,639	—	—	2,978,564	4,702,396
2007	1,868,643	1,463,661	—[e]	—[e]	3,307,691	4,790,858
2008	1,911,986	1,483,423	—[e]	—[e]	3,095,246	4,876,973
2009	1,945,531	1,500,044	—[e]	—[e]	3,151,284	4,960,643

The Indian Health Service (IHS): An Overview 27

Year	Indian Health Service (IHS)		Bureau of Indian Affairs (BIA)[a]		Census Bureau	
	Service Population (in IHS service areas; est.)	User Population (at IHS facilities)	Service Population (on or near reservations; est.)[b]	Tribal Enrollment (national; est.)	American Indian/Alaska Native race alone (est.)[c]	American Indian/Alaska Native Race Alone or in Combination with Other Races (est.)[d]
2010	1,981,213	1,524,346	—e	—e	Decennial: 3,739,507	Decennial: 5,220,579
2011	2,016,143	1,542,164	—e	—e	3,814,772	
2012	2,051,718	1,561,075	—e	—e	—	—

Sources: *IHS user and service population data*—IHS, *Trends in Indian Health* and *Regional Differences in Indian Health* both authored by U.S. Department of Health and Human Services, Public Health Service, Indian Health Service, Office of Planning, Evaluation, and Legislation, Division of Program Statistics, and published in Rockville, MD, and IHS, personal communication, August 13, 2013. *BIA service population*—1991: *Indian Service Population and Labor Force Estimates* (1991), Table 1 (recalculated by CRS). BIA service population and tribal enrollment, 1997: *Indian Labor Force Report: Portrait 1997*, "National Totals" table. BIA service population and tribal enrollment, 1999: *Indian Labor Force Report, 1999*, "National Totals" table. BIA service population and tribal enrollment, 2001: *Indian Labor Force Report, 2001*, "National Totals" table. BIA service population and tribal enrollment, 2003: *Indian Labor Force Report, 2003*, "National Totals" table. BIA service population and tribal enrollment, 2005: *Indian Labor Force Report, 2005*, "National Totals" table. All BIA publications are authored by U.S. Department of the Interior, Bureau of Indian Affairs, and published in Washington, D.C. *Census Bureau*—U.S. Bureau of the Census, (July 1): *Population Estimates,* http://www.census.gov/popest/data/historical/index. html. For 2000 and 2010 data: Tina Norris, Paula L. Winves, and Elizabeth M. Hoeffel, *The American Indian and Alaska Native Population:2010*, U.S. Department of Commerce, Economics and Statistics Administration, U.S. Census Bureau, 2010 Census Briefs, Washington, DC, January 2012.

[a] 2005 is the most recent year of the BIA data released. The BIA attempted to survey the tribes in 2010 about their service population and labor force estimates, but due to methodological concerns, these data were never released. See Letter from Donald E. Laverdure, Acting Assistant Secretary of Indian Affairs, to Tribal Leader, July 2, 2012, http://www.bia.gov/cs/groups/public/documents /text/idc-019173.pdf.

[b] The Bureau of Indian Affairs defines "near reservation" as areas or communities either contiguous or adjacent to a reservation that are so designated by the Department's Interior's Assistant Secretary of the Interior for Indians Affairs.

These areas are so designated, in consultation with the relevant Indian Tribe or Alaska Native village governing body, based on criteria such as the number of American Indians or Alaska Natives residing in the area, whether these residents have close affiliation with the Indian Tribe or reservation, the proximity of the area to the reservation, and whether BIA will be able to provide services to this area.

c Census data are estimates except in decennial Census years (2000 and 2010).

d Census data are estimates except in decennial Census years (2000 and 2010). The Census Bureau only began collecting data on American Indians alone or in combination with another race in the 2000 Census.

e The BIA has not released its Indian Labor Force Report since 2005.

While IHS, Census, and BIA figures for Indians, whether resident in urban areas or not, may not be definitive for the IHS-eligible population, they provide useful approximations of the population that IHS serves. Census data suggest that most American Indians/Alaska Natives live outside reservations and other census-identified Indian areas, that the movement out of these areas is many decades old, and that a majority of census-identified Indians live in census-identified urban areas.[107]

Many urban areas are within IHS service delivery areas, so further analysis may be needed to determine what proportion of census-identified urban Indians are eligible for general IHS services.

APPENDIX B. BRIEF HISTORY OF FEDERAL INVOLVEMENT IN INDIAN HEALTH

The following timeline (see **Figure B-1** and **Figure B-2**) presents a brief overview of federal involvement in Indian health. Federal involvement began as infectious disease control (e.g., smallpox vaccines), but grew over time to encompass more services and eventually evolved into the modern day IHS. Federal involvement in Indian health is rooted in treaties between Indian Tribes and the federal government. Over time, federal involvement has been formalized in legislation.

The timeline below presents some selected events both Indian health specific and some related historical events to provide context. The timeline is followed by a more detailed list of sources.

The Indian Health Service (IHS): An Overview

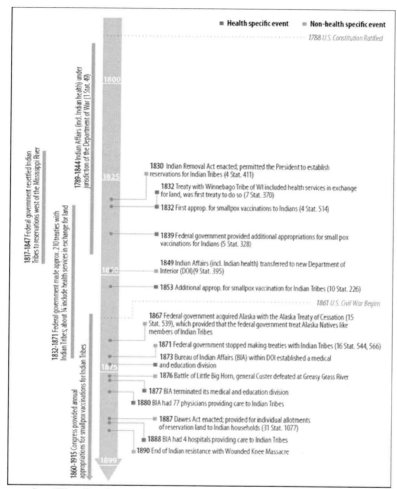

Sources: See "Timeline Sources" section below. Some information in this timeline was adapted from an archived CRS report authored by Roger Walke, former CRS Specialist in American Indian Policy.

Figure B-1. Brief Timeline of Federal Involvement in Indian Health (Part 1).

30   Elayne J. Heisler

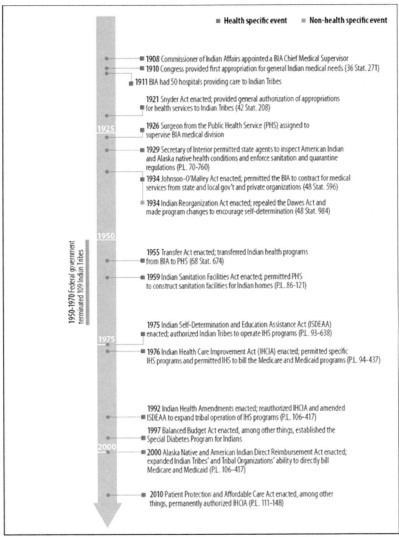

Sources: See "Timeline Sources" section below. Some information in this timeline was adapted from an archived CRS report authored by Roger Walke, former CRS Specialist in American Indian Policy.

Figure B-2. Brief Timeline of Federal Involvement in Indian Health (Part 2).

The Indian Health Service (IHS): An Overview 31

TIMELINE SOURCES

Dix, Mim and Yvette Roubideaux (ed) *Promises to Keep: Public Health Policy for American Indians and Alaska Natives in the 21st Century*, ed. (Washington, DC: American Public Health Association, 2001).

Kappler, Charles J., comp. *Indian Affairs: Laws and Treaties*, 7 vols. (Washington: GPO, 1904- [1979]).

Pfefferbaum, Betty, et al. "Learning How to Heal: An Analysis of the History, Policy, and Framework of Indian Health Care," *American Indian Law Review*, vol. 20, no. 2, 1995-1996, pp. 365-397.

Prucha, Francis Paul. *The Great Father: The United States Government and the American Indians* (Lincoln: University of Nebraska Press, 1984).

Schmeckebier, Laurence F. *The Office of Indian Affairs: Its History, Activities, and Organization* (Baltimore: Johns Hopkins Press, 1927).

Stuart, Paul. *Nations Within a Nation, Historical Statistics of American Indians* (New York, Greenwood Press, 1987).

U.S. American Indian Policy Review Commission, Task Force Six: Indian Health, *Report on Indian Health. Final Report to the American Indian Policy Review Commission*, July 1976 (Washington: GPO, 1978).

U.S. Congress. House of Representatives. Committee on Energy and Commerce. Subcommittee on Health and the Environment. *Indian Health Care: An Overview of the Federal Government's Role*, 98th Cong., 2nd sess. H.Prt. 98-Y, April 1984 (Washington: GPO, 1984).

CRS Report R41630, *The Indian Health Care Improvement Act Reauthorization and Extension as Enacted by the ACA: Detailed Summary and Timeline*, by Elayne J. Heisler.

End Notes

[1] Section 3 of the Indian Health Care Improvement Act (P.L. 94-437, 25 U.S.C. §1602).

[2] See Felix S. Cohen, *Felix S. Cohen's Handbook of Federal Indian Law* (1982 edition), Rennard Strickland, editor-inchief (Charlottesville, VA: Michie Bobbs-Merrill, 1982), p. 677; and Felix S. Cohen, *Cohen's Handbook of Federal Indian Law* (2005 edition), Nell Jessup Newton, editor-in-chief (Newark, NJ: LexisNexis [Matthew Bender & Company], 2005), §22.01(3).

[3] 25 U.S.C. §§1601 et seq; permanently authorized in §102201 of P.L. 111-148, as amended; for more detailed information see CRS Report R41630, *The Indian Health Care Improvement Act Reauthorization and Extension as Enacted by the ACA: Detailed Summary and Timeline*.

32   Elayne J. Heisler

[4] Certain other American Indians and Alaska Natives, including urban Indians, may also be eligible for health services at IHS-funded facilities. (See report section "IHS Eligibility").

[5] P.L. 93-638, as amended; 25 U.S.C. §450 et seq.

[6] U.S. Department of Health and Human Services, Indian Health Service, "Tribal Self-Governance," January 2013, http://www.ihs.gov/newsroom/factsheets/tribalselfgovernance/.

[7] In FY2013, IHS received appropriations under P.L. 112-175 and P.L. 113-6.

[8] The history of this appropriation and current authorized funding are described in CRS Report R42944, *Medicare, Medicaid, and Other Health Provisions in the American Taxpayer Relief Act of 2012*, coordinated by Jim Hahn.

[9] Diabetes funding and collections will be discussed later in this report. For information on total funding, see U.S. Dept. of Health and Human Services, Indian Health Service, *Fiscal Year 2014 Indian Health Service Justification of Estimates*, http://www.ihs.gov/BudgetFormulation/documents/FY2014BudgetJustification.pdf; hereinafter, *FY2014 IHS Budget Justification*. See also, IHS FY2013 SequestrationOperating Plan at http://www.ihs.gov/BudgetFormulation/documents/IHSFY2013 OperatingPlan.pdf.

[10] For information about IHS eligibility, see report section "IHS Eligibility." IHS is statutorily prohibited from charging eligible American Indians and Alaska Natives for services (see 25 U.S.C.§1681 and 25 U.S.C. §458aaa-14), but 25 U.S.C. §1680r permits tribes providing IHS-funded services through an ISDEAA compact to bill American Indians and Alaska Natives. In addition, some urban programs may charge for services.

[11] Mark Carroll, "Innovation in Indian Healthcare: Using Health Information Technology to Achieve Health Equity for American Indian and Alaska Native Populations," *Perspectives in Health Information Management*, Winter 2011.

[12] This report does not discuss IHS funding. This information is available in CRS reports that discuss the Interior, Environment, and Related Agencies appropriations bills, see http://www.crs.gov/pages/subissue.aspx?   cliid=2346&   parentid=73&preview=False. Information on IHS funding from FY2010 through FY2013 and proposed funding for FY2014 can be found in CRS Report R43304, *Public Health Service Agencies: Overview and Funding*, coordinated by Amalia K. Corby-Edwards and C. Stephen Redhead.

[13] IHS, personal communication, August 13, 2013.

[14] For information about American Indians and Alaska Natives who self-identify in the Census, see Tina Norris, Paula L. Winves, and Elizabeth M. Hoeffel, *The American Indian and Alaska Native Population:2010*, U.S. Department of Commerce, Economics and Statistics Administration, U.S. Census Bureau, 2010 Census Briefs, Washington, DC, January 2012.

[15] For example, P.L. 95-375 recognized the Pascua Yaqui Tribe of Arizona and set certain membership criteria.

[16] 42 C.F.R. §136.12(a). The Bureau of Indian Affairs (BIA) is an agency within the U.S. Department of the Interior.

[17] 25 U.S.C. §1680c: Health Services for Ineligible Persons.

[18] 25 U.S.C. §§1603(f), 1651-1660d.

[19] U.S. Government Accountability Office, *Indian Health Service: Action Needed to Ensure Equitable Allocation of Resources for the Contract Health Service Program*, 12-446, June 2012, http://www.gao.gov/assets/600/591631.pdf.

[20] FY2014 IHS Budget Justification.

[21] IHS user and service population data from IHS, personal communication, August 13, 2013.

[22] CRS Report R40551, *The 2010 Decennial Census: Background and Issues*, by Jennifer D. Williams.

The Indian Health Service (IHS): An Overview 33

[23] Indian Health Service (IHS) Statistical Note, "Department of Health and Human Services, Indian Health Service," press release, April 8, 1993, http://www.ihs.gov/california/assets/File/Training/Defining IHSPopulationEs.pdf.

[24] The 2010 IHCIA reauthorization required that IHS develop a plan to create a new Nevada area office. This office is not yet established, but should this occur, IHS would have 13 area offices. See discussion of the reauthorization of the Indian Health Care Improvement Act in CRS Report R41630, *The Indian Health Care Improvement Act Reauthorization and Extension as Enacted by the ACA: Detailed Summary and Timeline*, by Elayne J. Heisler.

[25] FY2014 IHS Budget Justification.

[26] Although the California area office covers most of California, some counties in California are covered by both the California area office and the Phoenix area office.

[27] P.L. 93-638, act of January 4, 1975, 88 Stat. 2203, as amended; 25 U.S.C. 450 et seq.

[28] U.S. Department of Health and Human Services, Indian Health Service, "Tribal Self-Governance," January 2013, http://www.ihs.gov/newsroom/factsheets/tribalselfgovernance/.

[29] Tribes that are served by IHS-operated facilities are sometimes referred to as "direct service tribes."

[30] CRS analysis of FY2014 IHS Budget Justification.

[31] CRS Analysis of IHS FY2012 user population data, and information from the IHS Office of Congressional and Legislative Affairs, August 13, 2013.

[32] FY2014 IHS Budget Justification.

[33] FY2014 IHS Budget Justification.

[34] Department of Health and Human Services, Indian Health Service, Division of Behavioral Health, "Fact Sheet: Youth Regional Treatment Centers,"http://www.ihs.gov/Behavioral/documents/yrtc-fact-sheet.pdf.

[35] 42 U.S.C. §254b.

[36] For more information on federal health center grants, see CRS Report R42433, *Federal Health Centers*, by Elayne J. Heisler.

[37] U.S. Government Accountability Office, *Indian Health Service: Health Care Services Are Not Always Available to Native Americans*, 05-789, August 31, 2005, http://www.gao.gov/assets/250/247558.pdf.

[38] Funding for urban programs is authorized under Title V of the Indian Health Care Improvement Act (25 U.S.C. 1651-1660h), which directs the HHS Secretary to make grants to or contracts with UIOs under the authority of the Snyder Act (25 U.S.C. 13). Such grants or contracts are not ISDEAA self-determination grants or contracts. See also, FY2014 IHS Budget Justification.

[39] FY2014 IHS Budget Justification.

[40] Ibid. Under Title V of the Indian Health Care Improvement Act, UIOs are not prohibited from charging their patients.

[41] See 42 CFR 136.11, "Services available."

[42] In statute, IHS is prohibited from using funds from its appropriation to perform abortions (25 U.S.C. §1676).

[43] FY2014 IHS Budget Justification.

[44] See Figure 2.

[45] FY2014 IHS Budget Justification.

[46] Scott Wetterhall et al., *Evaluation of the Dental Health Aide Therapist Workforce Model in Alaska: Final Report*, RTI International, Prepared for W.K. Kellogg Foundation, Rasmussen Foundation, and Bethel Community Services Foundation, Research Triangle Park, NC, October 2010.

[47] More information about these programs can be found in the following CRS reports: CRS Report R40425, *Medicare Primer*, coordinated by Patricia A. Davis and Scott R. Talaga; CRS Report RL33202, *Medicaid: A Primer*, by Elicia J. Herz; and CRS Report R42747, *Health Care for Veterans: Answers to Frequently Asked Questions*, by Sidath Viranga Panangala and Erin Bagalman.

[48] The ability to bill private insurance is not unique to IHS, but the ability to bill Medicare, Medicaid, CHIP, and the Department of Veterans Affairs is, as is the ability to retain reimbursements from federal sources to supplement the agency's appropriation. P.L. 94-437 at 25 U.S.C. §§1601 et seq.

[49] U.S. Department of Health and Human Services, Indian Health Service, "IHS Fact Sheet: Contract Health Services," January 2013, http://www.ihs.gov/newsroom/factsheets/contracthealthservices/. Some ITs and TOs use funds collected from Medicare, Medicaid, or other reimbursement sources to augment its PRC budget.

[50] 42 C.F.R. §136.23.

[51] 42 C.F.R. §136.61.

[52] IHS cannot require a beneficiary to enroll in an insurance program for which a beneficiary would be required to pay premiums.

[53] If an IT or a TO operates a PRC program, it will also use a medical priority system to determine if a PRC referral will be authorized.

[54] It may also be authorized to save a sense. For example, certain vision services are considered priority one because they are considered medically necessary to prevent blindness. If additional funds are available PRC may be authorized for additional priority levels of care.

[55] Thirty days for disabled individuals and seniors (25 U.S.C. §1646). See 42 C.F.R. 136.24.

[56] 25 U.S.C.§1621u.

[57] This requirement was included in Section 508 of the Medicare Modernization Act (P.L. 108-173).

[58] U.S. Government Accountability Office, *Indian Health Service: Capping Payments for Nonhospital Services Could Save Millions of Dollars for Contract Health Services*, 13-272, April 11, 2013, http://www.gao.gov/products/GAO-13 272.

[59] FY2014 IHS Budget Justification.

[60] U.S. Department of Health and Human Services, Indian Health Service, "IHS Fact Sheet: Diabetes," January 2013, http://www.ihs.gov/newsroom/factsheets/diabetes/.

[61] FY2014 IHS Budget Justification.

[62] Ibid.

[63] Department of Health and Human Services, Indian Health Service, "For American Indian and Alaska Native Youth," http://www.ihs.gov/Behavioral/documents/strengthen-factsheet.pdf.and FY2014 IHS Budget Justification.

[64] See Department of Health and Human Services, Indian Health Service, "Behavioral Health," http://www.ihs.gov/ Behavioral/ and CRS Report R41630, *The Indian Health Care Improvement Act Reauthorization and Extension as Enacted by the ACA: Detailed Summary and Timeline*, by Elayne J. Heisler Act Reauthorization and Extension as Enacted by the ACA: Detailed Summary and Timeline, by Elayne J. Heisler.

[65] FY2014 IHS Budget Justification.

[66] Ibid.

[67] The Alaska Native Tribal Health Consortium is a TO that represents a consortium of Alaska Native villages.

[68] P.L. 86-121, act of July 31, 1959, 73 Stat. 267; 42 U.S.C. 2004a.

The Indian Health Service (IHS): An Overview 35

[69] U.S. Department of Health and Human Services, Indian Health Service, "IHS Fact Sheets: Safe Water and Waste Disposal Facilities," January 2013, http://www.ihs.gov/newsroom/factsheets/safewater/.

[70] Ibid.

[71] Unless otherwise noted this section is drawn from the FY2014 IHS Budget Justification.

[72] The Joint Commission accredits and certifies health care organizations to ensure that certain standards are met. See http://www.jointcommission.org/about_us/about_the_joint_commission_main.aspx.

[73] For example, health centers, which are also located in rural or otherwise underserved areas also have provider vacancies. For discussion of these facilities, see CRS Report R42433, *Federal Health Centers*, by Elayne J. Heisler.

[74] U.S. Congress, Senate Indian Affairs, *Statement of Yvette Roubideaux, Acting Director, Indian Health Service*, Nomination Hearing for the Director of the Indian Health Service, 113th Cong., 1st sess., June 12, 2013.

[75] IHCIA §104 (25 U.S.C. §1613a).

[76] IHCIA §108 (U.S.C.§1616a-1).

[77] IHCIA §116 (25 U.S.C. §1616i).

[78] U.S. Department of Health and Human Services, *FY 2014 Budget in Brief*, Washington, DC, February 2013, http://www.hhs.gov/budget/fy2014/fy-2014-budget-in-brief.pdf.

[79] 25 U.S.C. §450 et seq.

[80] See U.S. General Accounting Office, *Indian Self-Determination Act: Shortfalls in Indian Contract Support Costs Need to Be Addressed*, GAO/RCED-99-150, June 1999, http://www.gao.gov/archive/1999/rc99150.pdf.

[81] *Salazar v. Ramah Navajo*, No. 11-551, slip op. (June 18, 2012), available at http://www.supremecourt.gov/opinions/ 11pdf/11-551.pdf and CRS Report WSLG119, *Supreme Court Holds the Government Liable for Contract Support Costs in Indian Self-Determination Contracts Even When Congress Fails to Appropriate Adequate Funds*, by Jane M. Smith.

[82] FY2014 IHS Budget Justification.

[83] P.L. 67-85, 42 Stat. 208, as amended; 25 U.S.C. §13.

[84] P.L. 83-568, act of August 5, 1954, 68 Stat. 674, as amended; 42 U.S.C. §2001 et seq.

[85] There is some evidence that HHS was better suited to administer the agency, because after the IHS was transferred to HHS, IHS began to construct facilities on or near reservations, and the rate of deaths for a number of conditions including tuberculosis, influenza, and pneumonia declined. It is not possible to directly attribute these declines (either partially or entirely) to the transfer. *Promises to Keep: Public Health Policy for American Indians and Alaska Natives in the 21st Century*, ed. Mim Dixon and Yvette Roubideaux (Washington, DC: American Public Health Association, 2001).

[86] P.L. 86-121, act of July 31, 1959, 73 Stat. 267; 42 U.S.C. §2004a.

[87] FY2014 IHS Budget Justification.

[88] P.L. 93-638, act of January 4, 1975, 88 Stat. 2203, as amended; 25 U.S.C. §§450 et seq.

[89] P.L. 94-437, act of September 30, 1976, 90 Stat. 1400, as amended; 25 U.S.C.§§1601 et seq., and 42 U.S.C. §1395qq, 1396j (and amending other sections).

[90] P.L. 102-573, act of October 29, 1992, 106 Stat. 4526. Previous reauthorizations occurred in 1980 (P.L. 96-537) and 1988 (P.L. 100-713), and substantial amendments were made in 1990 (P.L. 101-630, Title V).

[91] Omnibus Indian Advancement Act, P.L. 106-568, §815, act of December 27, 2000, 114 Stat. 2868, 2918.

[92] P.L. 111-148, as amended.

[93] P.L. 102-573, act of October 29, 1992, 106 Stat. 4526, 4590.

[94] Title II of P.L. 100-472, act of October 5, 1988, 102 Stat. 2285, 2296.

[95] P.L. 106-260, act of August 18, 2000, 114 Stat. 711; 25 U.S.C. §458aaa et seq.

[96] P.L. 106-417, act of November 1, 2000, 114 Stat.1812; 25 U.S.C §1645 and 1601 note, and 42 U.S.C. 1395qq(e), 1396j(d).

[97] §10221 of P.L. 111-148.

[98] CRS Report R41630, *The Indian Health Care Improvement Act Reauthorization and Extension as Enacted by the ACA: Detailed Summary and Timeline*, by Elayne J. Heisler.

[99] CRS Report R41152, *Indian Health Care: Impact of the Affordable Care Act (ACA)*, by Elayne J. Heisler.

[100] The Census allows respondents to identify their tribe, but this is still self-identification. The Census does not confirm a respondent's enrollment (or eligibility) in a federally recognized tribe.

[101] The Census Bureau also collects population data through the American Community Survey an ongoing survey that includes population estimates based on three-year averages. For a description of the American Community Survey see http://www.census.gov/acs/www/about_the_survey/american_community_survey/ and CRS Report R41532, *The American Community Survey: Development, Implementation, and Issues for Congress*, by Jennifer D. Williams.

[102] Tina Norris, Paula L. Winves, and Elizabeth M. Hoeffel, *The American Indian and Alaska Native Population:2010*, U.S. Department of Commerce, Economics and Statistics Administration, U.S. Census Bureau, 2010 Census Briefs, Washington, DC, January 2012.

[103] U.S. Department of Health and Human Services, Indian Health Service, Office of Public Health, Division of Community and Environmental Health, Program Statistics Team, *Regional Differences in Indian Health, 1998-99* (Rockville, MD: IHS, 2000), p. 11.

[104] See discussion in "IHS Service Population."

[105] U.S. Department of the Interior, Bureau of Indian Affairs, Office of Tribal Services, *Indian Labor Force Report, 1999* (Washington: BIA, n.d.), pp. I-iii.

[106] See 25 U.S.C. 1603(f), 1651 *et seq.*

[107] Ralph Forquera, *Urban Indian Health*, The Henry J. Kaiser Family Foundation, Issue Brief, Washington, DC, November 2001, p. 1 and Appendix 1, http://kaiserfamily foundation.files.wordpress.com/2001/10/ 6326urbanindianhealth.pdf; and Marlita A. Reddy ed., *Statistical Record of Native North Americans* (Detroit: Gale Research, 1993), p. 420.

In: The Indian Health Service
Editor: Pamela M. Agnelli

ISBN: 978-1-63321-582-5
© 2014 Nova Science Publishers, Inc.

Chapter 2

INDIAN HEALTH SERVICE: OPPORTUNITIES MAY EXIST TO IMPROVE THE CONTRACT HEALTH SERVICES PROGRAM[*]

United States Government Accountability Office

WHY GAO DID THIS STUDY

IHS provides health care to American Indians and Alaska Natives. When services are unavailable from IHS, IHS's CHS program may pay for care from external providers. GAO previously reported on challenges regarding the timeliness of CHS payments and the number of American Indians and Alaska Natives who may gain new health care coverage as a result of PPACA. PPACA mandated GAO to review the CHS program. This report examines (1) the length of time it takes external providers to receive payment from IHS after delivering CHS services; (2) the performance measures IHS has established for processing CHS provider payments; (3) the factors that affect the length of time it takes IHS to pay CHS providers; and (4) how new PPACA health care coverage options could affect the program. To conduct this work, GAO analyzed fiscal year 2011 CHS claims data, interviewed IHS officials, including officials in four IHS areas, and reviewed agency documents and statutes.

---

[*] This is an edited, reformatted and augmented version of a United States Government Accountability Office publication, No. GAO-14-57, dated December 2013.

WHAT GAO RECOMMENDS

GAO recommends that IHS revise an agency measure of the timeliness with which purchase orders are issued, use available funds as appropriate to improve the alignment between CHS staffing levels and workloads, and proactively develop potential options to streamline CHS eligibility requirements. The agency concurred with two recommendations, but did not concur with the recommendation to use available funds to improve CHS staffing levels. GAO believes the recommendation is valid as discussed in the report.

WHAT GAO FOUND

For Indian Health Service (IHS) contract health services (CHS) delivered in fiscal year 2011, a majority of claims were paid within 6 months of the service delivery date, but some took much longer. Specifically, about 73 percent of claims were paid within 6 months of service delivery, while about 8 percent took more than 1 year. The CHS payment process consists of three main steps: (1) the local CHS program issues a purchase order to the provider authorizing payment (either before service delivery, or after, such as in emergency situations), (2) the provider submits a claim for payment, and (3) IHS pays the provider. GAO found that the first step took the longest—often taking more than 2 months.

IHS uses three measures to assess the time it takes to approve and then process payments to CHS providers. Two of the measures concern the first step in the payment process (purchase order issuance) and the third concerns the final step (making the payment). One of the measures IHS uses to assess the timeliness of the first step is the average time it takes to issue a purchase order after a service has been delivered; IHS's current target for this measure is 74 days. However, the measure does not provide a clear picture of timeliness for this activity as it combines data for two different types of CHS services—those for which payment eligibility was determined prior to service delivery and those for which eligibility was determined after service delivery. IHS officials told GAO that when eligibility is determined prior to service delivery, it may take only one day from the date of service to issue the purchase order. Including this type of service in the calculation, therefore, lowers the overall average.

The complexity of the CHS program affects the timeliness of provider payments. IHS program officials make decisions on what care will be funded on a case-bycase basis, evaluating each case against a number of eligibility requirements involving multiple steps. This process can lead to payment delays. Officials noted that delays also can occur when processing payments and that staffing shortages can affect the timeliness of payments. Some program officials noted that their staffing levels were below standards established by IHS.

New coverage options in the Patient Protection and Affordable Care Act (PPACA) may provide an opportunity to simplify CHS eligibility requirements. PPACA made significant changes to the Medicaid program and included new health care coverage options that may benefit many American Indians and Alaska Natives beginning in 2014. IHS officials reported the agency developed the current CHS program eligibility requirements to manage CHS program funding constraints. In particular, some of the complexities of the program were designed to allow the program to operate within the constrained levels of program funding. With the availability of new coverage options under PPACA, some constraints on CHS program funds could be alleviated, providing IHS an opportunity to streamline service eligibility requirements and expand the range of services it pays for with CHS funds.

ABBREVIATIONS

CHS	contract health services
CHSDA	contract health service delivery area
FI	fiscal intermediary
GPRA	Government Performance Results Act
HHS	Department of Health and Human Services
HIS	Indian Health Service
PPACA	Patient Protection and Affordable Care Act of 2010

December 11, 2013

Congressional Addressees

The Indian Health Service (IHS), an agency within the Department of Health and Human Services (HHS), is charged with providing health care

40   United States Government Accountability Office

services to the approximately 2.1 million American Indians and Alaska Natives who are members or descendants of federally recognized tribes.[1] These services are provided at federally or tribally operated health care facilities,[2] which receive IHS funding and are located in 12 federally designated geographic areas overseen by IHS area offices.[3] These facilities vary in the services they are able to provide; for example, some facilities offer comprehensive hospital services, while others offer only primary care services. When services are not available at these facilities, the facilities may use IHS's contract health services (CHS) program funds to obtain care for eligible patients from external health care providers, including hospitals and office-based physicians.

At the local level, the CHS program is administered by individual CHS programs generally affiliated with IHS-funded facilities. IHS has oversight authority over local CHS programs that are affiliated with IHS-operated facilities.[4] The local CHS programs determine whether to pay for services from external providers based on requirements that are unique to CHS.

This report is one in a series of reports we have conducted in the last 3 years that have examined the CHS program.[5] In our previous reports, we identified challenges cited by providers with the CHS program payment process.[6] We found, for example, that according to providers, sometimes it took months or years to receive payment after providing a service, which added to the burden of both patients and providers.[7] In addition, we reported on the number of American Indians and Alaska Natives who may gain new health care coverage beginning in 2014[8] as a result of provisions in the Patient Protection and Affordable Care Act (PPACA) of 2010.[9]

PPACA mandated GAO to examine the administration of the CHS program.[10] This report focuses on the timeliness of CHS payments to providers and how changes in PPACA could affect the CHS program. Specifically, this report examines:

1) the length of time it takes external providers to receive payment from IHS after delivering CHS services;
2) the performance measures that IHS has established for the amount of time it takes to process CHS provider payments;
3) the factors that affect the length of time it takes IHS to pay CHS providers; and
4) how new health care coverage options included in PPACA could affect the CHS program.

To determine the length of time after service delivery that payments are made, we obtained IHS data on paid CHS claims for health care services delivered in fiscal year 2011 that were authorized by IHS-operated CHS programs in 10 areas and that were paid as of February 2013; a total of approximately 398,000 claims.[11] Claims data from fiscal year 2011 were the most recent sufficiently complete data available for our analysis. We assessed the reliability of IHS's federal CHS program claims data by reviewing documentation and discussing the data with knowledgeable officials. We also performed data reliability checks, such as examining the data for missing values and obvious errors, to test the internal consistency and reliability of the data. We determined that the data were sufficiently reliable for our purposes.

To examine IHS's performance measures for the amount of time it takes IHS-operated CHS programs to process provider payments, we reviewed relevant statutes, agency documentation, and interviewed officials from IHS headquarters, areas, and CHS programs.

To determine the factors that affect the length of time to pay providers, we interviewed IHS officials in selected areas and CHS programs. We conducted interviews in four areas: Albuquerque, Billings, Navajo, and Oklahoma; and within each of these areas, at three local IHS-operated CHS programs. We selected these 4 areas and 12 programs to reflect a range in the length of time for paying CHS claims based on previous claims data. In our interviews, we asked officials about their procedures for processing CHS referrals and the factors they believed affected the length of time to pay providers. In addition, we interviewed IHS's fiscal intermediary, who is responsible for the final processing of payments to providers. We also reviewed relevant statutes and agency regulations and documentation.

To determine the effect that new coverage options available in PPACA might have on the CHS program, we reviewed relevant statutes and our recent report on eligibility among American Indian and Alaska Natives for new coverage options available in PPACA.[12]

We conducted this performance audit from November 2012 to November 2013 in accordance with generally accepted government auditing standards. Those standards require that we plan and perform the audit to obtain sufficient, appropriate evidence to provide a reasonable basis for our findings and conclusions based on our audit objectives. We believe that the evidence obtained provides a reasonable basis for our findings and conclusions based on our audit objectives.

42 United States Government Accountability Office

BACKGROUND

CHS Program Organization

IHS facilities and their associated CHS programs are located in 12 geographic areas, each overseen by an IHS area office led by an Area Director. Ten of the 12 areas include at least some IHS-operated facilities; these 10 areas oversee local CHS programs in 33 states. IHS headquarters sets CHS program policies and oversees the areas. Each IHS area contains multiple local CHS programs. The areas distribute funds to the local CHS programs in their areas, monitor the programs, and establish procedures and provide guidance and technical assistance to the programs.

CHS Program Funding and Service Eligibility Requirements

The CHS program is funded through annual appropriations and must operate within the limits of available appropriated funds.[13] Based on the regulations that IHS has established for the CHS program, a number of requirements must be met in order for a service to be eligible for CHS payment.[14] Based on the requirements, before approving a service for payment, local CHS programs must consider the following:

- **Is the patient a member or descendent of a federally recognized tribe or someone with close ties to the tribe?** To be eligible for CHS payment, the service must be for a patient who is a member or descendent of a federally recognized tribe or someone who maintains close economic and social ties with the tribe.
- **Does the patient reside within the Tribal Contract Health Service Delivery Area (CHSDA)?** For a service to be paid for with CHS funds, it must be for a patient who resides in the Tribal CHSDA. Unless otherwise established, the CHSDA encompasses the reservation, the counties that border the reservation, and other specified lands.[15] Exceptions exist for students who are temporarily absent from their CHSDA during full-time study and individuals who are temporarily absent from the CHSDA for less than 180 days due to travel or employment.
- **Are alternate health care resources available to the patient?** Many users of IHS services are also eligible for other sources of payment for

care, including Medicaid, Medicare, and private insurance.[16] The CHS program is typically the payer of last resort.[17] Therefore, before a service is approved for CHS payment, the patient must apply for and use all alternate resources that are available and accessible. Services from an IHS facility are also considered a resource, so CHS funds cannot be used for services reasonably accessible and available at IHS facilities.

- **Did the CHS program receive timely notification of services provided from a non-IHS facility?** In non-emergency cases, the local CHS program should be notified and the service approved for payment prior to the patient receiving care. In cases where the patient was not referred for care by an IHS provider, such as with emergency room services, the CHS program must be notified within 72 hours of when the service was delivered. Notification may be made by the individual, provider, hospital, or someone on behalf of the individual in order for the service to be eligible for CHS payment. The notification time is extended to 30 days for the elderly and disabled.

- **Are the services considered medically necessary and listed as one of the established area medical or dental priorities?** To be eligible for payment under the CHS program, the service must be considered medically necessary and listed as one of the established IHS area's medical or dental priorities. A program committee that is part of the local CHS program evaluates the medical necessity of the service, for example, at a weekly meeting. IHS has established four broad medical priority levels of health care services eligible for payment and a fifth for excluded services that cannot be paid for with CHS program funds. Each area is required to establish priorities that are consistent with IHS's medical priority levels and are adapted to the specific needs of the CHS programs in its area. CHS programs that are affiliated with IHS-operated facilities must assign a priority level to services based on the priority system established by their area offices. Funds permitting, these CHS programs first pay for the highest priority services and then for all or some of the lower priority services they fund.[18] Our prior work has found that available CHS program funds have not been sufficient to pay for all eligible services.[19] At some IHS facilities, the amount of CHS funding available was only sufficient to cover cases with the highest medical priority—Priority 1—emergent or acutely urgent care services that are necessary to

44 United States Government Accountability Office

prevent immediate death or serious impairment of health. (See table 1 for a description of the medical priority levels and related services.)

Table 1. IHS Medical Priority Levels for Contract Health Services

Medical priority level	Services included in priority level
Level I	Emergent/acutely urgent care services, such as trauma care, acute/chronic renal replacement therapy, obstetrical delivery and neonatal care.
Level II	Preventive care services, such as preventive ambulatory care, routine prenatal care, and screening mammograms.
Level III	Primary and secondary care services, such as scheduled ambulatoryservices for nonemergent conditions, elective surgeries, and specialty consultations.
Level IV	Chronic tertiary and extended care services, such as rehabilitation care, skilled nursing facility care, and organ transplants.
Level V	Excluded services, such as cosmetic plastic surgery and experimental procedures that programs may not pay for with CHS program funds.

Source: GAO analysis of IHS documents.

After considering these questions, local CHS programs review each case based on the availability of funding and may defer or deny requests to pay for services when program funds are not available. If the CHS program determines that a service can be funded, it issues a purchase order for the service.

CHS Payment Process

In general, three entities are involved in the CHS payment process: (1) the local CHS program, (2) the provider, and (3) IHS's fiscal intermediary (FI). The timing of the CHS program's and the provider's involvement depends on whether the service was prompted by a referral from an IHS provider prior to the date of service—called IHS referrals, or prompted by the patient seeking care without first obtaining a referral from an IHS provider—these are typically emergency services and called self-referrals.

IHS Referrals

IHS referrals are cases in which an IHS-funded provider refers a patient for care to an external provider. The local CHS program receives the referral and evaluates it against the eligibility requirements. Once the CHS program receives the needed information to make its determination, it will:

- approve the service for payment and issue a purchase order to obligate the funds and send copies of the purchase order to the provider and to the FI;
- defer funding if it meets all the eligibility criteria, but funds are not available; or
- deny the service.

If the service is approved, the local CHS program typically works with an external provider to set up an appointment for the patient to receive the service and issues the purchase order to the provider—either before the service is provided or shortly after the service is provided. After performing the service, the external provider submits the purchase order along with the claim for payment to the FI. Once the FI receives the claim and purchase order from the external provider, it verifies the purchase order and patient data, evaluates whether alternate resources are available, and, if appropriate, makes the required payment. If there are any issues with the claim, such as missing information from the CHS program or provider, the FI will put the claim in a hold status until the issues are resolved.

Self-Referrals

Self-referrals are typically emergency situations where the patient receives services from external providers without first obtaining a referral from an IHS-funded provider. After the services are delivered, the provider seeks approval from the CHS program for payment for the services. With self-referrals, the steps taken by the CHS program to evaluate the referral against the program's eligibility requirements to determine whether the service is eligible for CHS payment do not begin until after the service is provided. In these cases, the local CHS program may have to communicate with the external provider, for example, requesting information about the services provided.

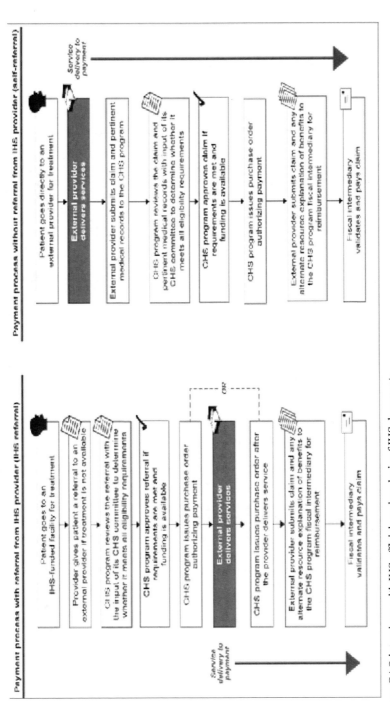

Source: GAO interviews with IHS officials and analysis of IHS documents.

Figure 1. Two Paths for Patient Care to Be Funded by Contract Health Services (CHS) Program.

Similar to IHS referrals, once the CHS program receives the needed information to make an eligibility determination, it will approve the service for payment and issue a purchase order to obligate the funds; defer funding the service; or deny the service. For approved self-referral services, once the FI receives the claim and purchase order from the external provider, it follows the same procedures for processing the payment as for IHS referrals. (See fig. 1 for an overview of the approval and payment processes for IHS referrals and self-referrals.)

For services that are ultimately paid for under the CHS program, whether they are IHS or self-referrals, the CHS payment process consists of three main steps that encompass the time from the date a service is delivered to the date the provider is paid.

1) **Local CHS program issues the purchase order.** The time for this step can be measured by the length of time between when a service is provided and when the local CHS program issues the purchase order. (Sometimes the purchase order is issued before the service is provided, such as for some IHS referrals; in these cases this step has no effect on the time it takes to pay the provider.)

2) **External provider submits a claim to IHS's FI.** The time for this step can be measured by the length of time between when the CHS program issues the purchase order and when the FI receives the claim.

3) **The FI pays the claim.** The time for this step can be measured by the length of time between when the FI receives a claim from an external provider and when the payment is made.

Health Care Coverage Options in PPACA Affecting American Indians and Alaska Natives

PPACA made significant changes to the Medicaid program and included new health care coverage options that may benefit American Indians and Alaska Natives. In 2014, Medicaid eligibility will expand in states opting to participate, such that all individuals with incomes at or below 138 percent of the federal poverty level will be eligible for the program, including previously ineligible categories of individuals, such as childless adults.[20] Also in 2014, health insurance exchanges will be available—health insurance marketplaces in which individuals and small businesses can compare, select, and purchase health coverage from participating carriers.[21] For individuals obtaining insurance through the exchanges, PPACA provides premium tax credits for those meeting certain income requirements and cost-sharing exemptions for qualifying American Indians and Alaska Natives.[22] Finally, in 2015, states may implement the new Basic Health Program option, under which the federal government will give states 95 percent of the premium tax credits and cost-sharing subsidies that would have been provided if the individuals had enrolled in the exchanges, to allow states to provide coverage for individuals with incomes between 138 and 200 percent of the federal poverty level.[23]

In previous work, we found that, after these changes are implemented many American Indians and Alaska Natives may gain new health care coverage options. For example, we estimated that more than half of American Indians and Alaska Natives may be eligible either for cost-sharing exemptions and premium tax credits for insurance obtained through the exchanges, or eligible for health care coverage through the new Basic Health Program or Medicaid, including those who are currently eligible for Medicaid but not enrolled, and those who will be newly eligible under 2014 eligibility rules. A significant proportion of American Indians and Alaska Natives reflected in this potential new enrollment live in IHS service areas.[24]

MORE THAN TWO-THIRDS OF CHS CLAIMS WERE PAID WITHIN 6 MONTHS BUT SOME TOOK MUCH LONGER TO PAY

For CHS services delivered in fiscal year 2011, a majority of providers' claims were paid within 6 months of the service delivery date, but some took much longer. More than one-third (38 percent) of claims processed by IHS-operated CHS programs were paid within 3 months after services were delivered. Another 35 percent were paid between 3 and 6 months of service delivery. The percentage of claims paid more than 6 months after service delivery was much smaller, with 19 percent of claims being paid between 6 months and 1 year after services were delivered, and about 8 percent paid more than 1 year after services were delivered. (See fig. 2.)

The amount of time it took to pay providers was not the same across all IHS areas. The areas varied in the amount of time between the date a service was provided and the date the claim was paid, particularly with respect to the percentage of claims that were paid within 3 months and within 6 months of service delivery. For example, although more than one-third of claims IHS-wide were paid within 3 months or less of service delivery, across IHS areas this percentage ranged from 18 percent in Albuquerque to 48 percent in Billings. Similarly, the percentage of claims paid within 6 months or less of service delivery ranged from 59 percent to 80 percent, also in Albuquerque and Billings, respectively. There was less variation among IHS areas in the percentage of claims paid within 1 year or less of service delivery, ranging from 87 percent in Albuquerque to 94 percent in Nashville. For 8 of the 10 IHS areas we reviewed, 90 percent or more of their claims were paid within 1 year of service delivery. (See fig. 3.)

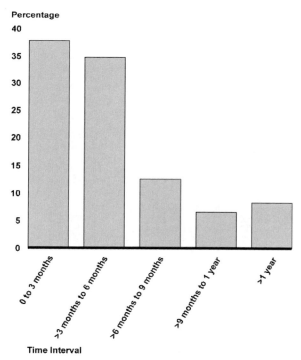

Source: GAO analysis of IHS claims data.
Note: Analysis was limited to claims processed by IHS-operated CHS programs and included all claims for services delivered in fiscal year 2011 that were paid as of February 2013.

Figure 2. Percentage of Contract Health Services (CHS) Claims Paid within Certain Time Intervals, for Services Delivered in Fiscal Year 2011.

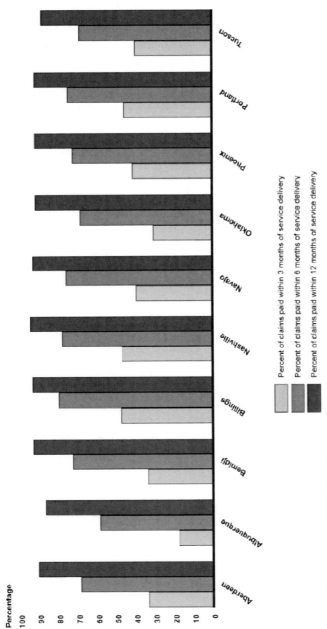

Source: GAO analysis of IHS claims data.

Note: Analysis was limited to claims processed by IHS-operated CHS programs and included all claims for services delivered in fiscal year 2011 that were paid as of February 2013.

Figure 3. Percentage of Contract Health Services (CHS) Claims Paid within 3 Months, 6 Months, and 1 Year of Service Delivery, for Services Delivered in Fiscal Year 2011, by IHS Area.

Indian Health Service 51

Among the three main steps in the payment process, the step that most often took the longest in the payment process was the first step—the time from date of service to the issuance of the purchase order. For services delivered in fiscal year 2011, purchase orders were issued in 1 month or less after services were delivered for 41 percent of claims. For another 40 percent of claims, purchase orders were issued more than 2 months after services were delivered; and in about half of these cases, the purchase order was issued more than 4 months after the service was delivered. In comparison, the second step—the time from the date the purchase order was issued to the date the FI received the claim from the provider—took 1 month or less for 61 percent of the services, and the third step—the time from the date the FI received the claim to the date payment was made—took 1 month or less for 83 percent of the claims. (See fig. 4.)

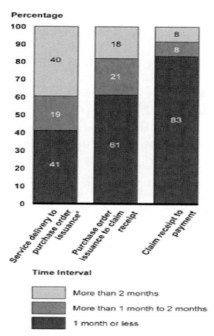

Source: GAO analysis of IHS claims data.
Notes: Analysis was limited to claims processed by IHS-operated CHS programs and included all claims for services delivered in fiscal year 2011 that were paid as of February 2013. Claims associated with purchase orders issued before the date of service were included in the analysis. Percentages may not add to 100 due to rounding.

52   United States Government Accountability Office

ªFor claims associated with purchase orders issued before the date of service, the timeframe from service delivery to purchase order was considered to be 1 month or less.

Figure 4. Percentage of Claims Processed within Certain Time Intervals in Each Step of the Contract Health Services (CHS) Payment Process, for Services Delivered in Fiscal Year 2011.

IHS HAS THREE TIMELINESS MEASURES FOR PROCESSING PROVIDER PAYMENTS, BUT THE TWO INVOLVING PURCHASE ORDER ISSUANCE DO NOT PROVIDE A CLEAR PICTURE OF TIMELINESS

IHS uses three measures to assess how long it takes to approve and then process payments to CHS providers. Two of these measures concern the first step in the payment process—the time it takes local CHS programs to approve payments to providers and issue purchase orders to them— but neither of these measures provides a clear or complete picture of the timeliness of these activities, which constitute the most time-consuming period within the provider payment process, according to our analyses. IHS also has a timeliness measure for the final step in the provider payment process—the time it takes IHS's FI to make payment to providers once it receives claims from them.[25] Descriptions of the three timeliness measures follow.

Government Performance Results Act (GPRA) Measure

The first of two measures that IHS uses to assess the timeliness of the first step in the provider payment process is the average time it takes for IHS to issue a purchase order after a service has been provided. IHS established this measure in fiscal year 2009 in response to GPRA, and has set annual targets for the measure since then. GPRA requires federal agencies to develop performance plans with annual goals and measures. (Hereafter, we refer to this as the GPRA measure.)

For fiscal years 2009 and 2010, IHS set the target for the GPRA measure at 82 days and 78 days, respectively. IHS missed the target by 28 days in 2009 and by 4 days in 2010. IHS kept the target at 78 days in fiscal year 2011, then lowered it to 74 days in 2012 and met these targets in both years. For fiscal year 2013, IHS kept the target at 74 days, and an IHS official said it would remain there for fiscal year 2014. According to IHS officials, the basis for the GPRA measure's target was a health care industry consultant's report showing average times that other health insurers, including private insurers and Medicaid, took to pay claims.

Although clear targets have been established for the GPRA measure, the way the measure is calculated does not result in a clear picture of whether the goal of the measure is being achieved. In our previous work, we found that successful performance metrics should demonstrate the degree to which desired results are achieved.[26] According to IHS, the goal of the GPRA measure is to decrease the average number of days from the provision of services to purchase order issuance. However, the GPRA measure does not provide a clear picture of the timeliness of purchase order issuance because it combines self-referrals with some IHS referrals when calculating the average time it takes for IHS to issue a purchase order, even though the timing of when purchase orders are issued relative to service delivery can be very different for the two referral types. The GPRA measure calculates the average time it takes to issue purchase orders for services for which the purchase order was issued after the service was provided. This includes all self-referrals, where none of the work to determine whether the service is eligible for CHS payment can be started before the service is delivered because IHS does not know about it until after the service has been delivered. However, it also includes some IHS referrals—referrals for which all of the work to determine whether the service is eligible for CHS payment generally is completed before the service is delivered. Some local CHS programs said they wait to issue purchase orders for IHS referrals until shortly after they confirm that the services were actually delivered. Officials from one local CHS program told us that for these referrals, it may take only one day from the date of service to issue the purchase order. Including these IHS referrals in the calculation of the GPRA measure gives an unclear picture of performance because the inclusion of IHS referrals lowers the overall GPRA average. IHS officials agreed that the calculation of the GPRA measure mixes IHS referrals with self-referrals, and CHS officials at one area office said the measure would be more useful if IHS and self-referrals were analyzed separately. However, IHS officials told us that because the agency's claims data system does not include a data field that tracks referral type, it does not have a way to separate the two different types of referrals that would allow the agency to systematically determine the average time it takes to issue purchase orders by referral type.

54   United States Government Accountability Office

IHS officials expressed varying opinions about the utility and quality of the GPRA measure. Some officials noted that before the measure was established, there was no timeliness performance measure for the CHS program. These officials told us that the measure has helped to identify local CHS programs that have implemented practices that help improve timeliness of payments. But officials also criticized the GPRA measure, noting that many of the factors that help to determine whether an area or local CHS program meets the target are not within the area's or the program's control, such as how quickly a program receives information from providers.

The Time It Takes to Make a Decision About a Claim

The other measure that IHS uses to assess the timeliness of the first step in the provider payment process is how long it takes from the time IHS is notified of a claim to when the agency makes a decision about it. Under a statutory provision, IHS must approve or deny the claim within 5 days of receiving "notification" of a provider's claim for a service or accept the claim as valid.[27] (Hereafter, we refer to this provision as the 5-day rule.) According to IHS officials, the agency has interpreted the rule's clock as beginning once a claim is "clean," or "completed," meaning that all information necessary to determine whether the claim should be approved, deferred, or denied has been obtained. IHS officials told us, however, that it is in obtaining this information—including medical records to determine medical priority and the availability of alternate resources—that delays most typically occur. Thus, the 5-day rule's clock does not begin until after completion of the part of the process in which IHS officials believe delays most typically occur. Although IHS officials said the agency's interpretation of the 5-day rule currently is not included in any official written guidance, they said the agency plans to include an explanation of its interpretation of the rule in revisions to the CHS chapter of the Indian Health Manual, which officials said is expected to be completed by early 2014.

The Time It Takes the FI to Pay the Claim

The third measure that IHS uses to assess the timeliness of the payment process focuses on the last step in the process—the length of time that the FI should take to process payments to providers once it receives claims from

Indian Health Service 55

them. IHS's contract with its FI specifies that at least 97 percent of clean claims are to be paid within 30 days of receiving the claim from the provider. Similar to the 5-day rule, the FI defines clean claims as those containing all required information, including the purchase order; passing all IHS and FI agreed-upon internal checks; and not requiring additional investigation by the FI. The FI issues monthly reports to IHS documenting its compliance with this provision. According to these reports, this target was met every month from January 2012 through July 2013.[28]

COMPLEXITY OF THE CHS PROGRAM, CHS STAFFING AND FUNDING AVAILABILITY, AND VARIATIONS IN PROGRAM PRACTICES CAN AFFECT THE TIMELINESS OF PAYMENTS TO PROVIDERS

The complex processes for determining whether a service is eligible for CHS funding can affect the timeliness of provider payments and result in delays. Even after a local CHS program determines that a service is eligible for CHS funding, complexities in the payment process managed by IHS's FI can result in delays. In addition, CHS officials reported that staffing shortages and limited funding contribute to delays in processing payments to providers. Local CHS programs also reported varying practices for assessing eligibility and approving CHS funding, which may contribute to variations in timeliness for provider payments.

Complex Processes for Determining Whether a Service Is Eligible for CHS Funding Can Affect the Timeliness of Provider Payments

IHS's process for determining whether services are eligible for CHS program funds is complex and different from processes used by other payers, which can affect the timeliness of provider payments. Unlike other payers that offer a defined set of benefits—including Medicare, Medicaid, and private insurers—the CHS program makes decisions about what care will be funded on a case-by-case basis, so that each time a referral for care is received by a local CHS program, it is evaluated against a number of eligibility requirements as well as against available funding. Evaluating a service against each of the

56 United States Government Accountability Office

service eligibility requirements involves multiple steps, some of which depend on the CHS program receiving information from providers, patients, and others, and delays can occur during the evaluation of some of these eligibility requirements, according to CHS officials. In some cases, making these eligibility determinations can be fairly involved, and can ultimately affect the amount of time it takes for a provider to receive payment after the service is delivered. The effects of this process on payment times is greater for self-referrals— situations in which the service was provided before it was approved for payment—because the entire process for determining whether the service was eligible for CHS payment does not begin until after the service was delivered. According to IHS officials, the agency developed the CHS program eligibility regulations in order to carefully manage and stretch limited CHS funding to provide the most critical services to the most patients.

Two aspects of the process for determining eligibility for CHS program funding were frequently reported as resulting in payment delays:

1) determining whether a service meets the area's medical priorities and
2) identifying all available alternate resources. Officials from 8 of 12 local CHS programs we interviewed reported payment delays related to determining whether a service met the area's medical priorities, and officials from 8 of 12 local CHS programs reported payment delays related to identifying all available alternate resources.

Determining medical priority can result in delays because local CHS programs must obtain from the provider medical records with sufficient detail to assess whether a service is medically necessary and falls within the established medical priorities. Officials reported that, while in some cases the necessary records have been provided relatively quickly (e.g., within a week) in other cases it has taken much longer. For example, some local CHS programs reported situations when it has taken weeks or months to obtain necessary medical documentation, and one program reported situations when it has taken as long as 1 to 2 years to receive this documentation. Program officials noted different reasons for these delays. For example, officials reported situations where providers have sent documentation to the wrong CHS program when the providers were unaware in which CHSDAs the patients resided. Another reason cited by local CHS program officials for delays in receipt of medical documentation included situations in which incomplete documentation was provided and the program needed to follow up with the provider.

Indian Health Service

57

Officials reported a number of situations in which determining whether the patient has alternate resources to pay for the service, has resulted in delays. For example, some local CHS program officials told us that when they believe a patient is eligible for alternate resources—such as Medicaid—they have the patient apply for those resources, and will hold off on approving a service for CHS funding until the determination is made on the application. Officials from one local CHS program said that Medicaid determinations in their state can sometimes take months. In another example, officials from one local CHS program stated that for situations involving car accidents or a fall on private property, determining liability can take a long time, and availability of alternate resources cannot be determined until decisions on liability have been determined. In another example, officials from one CHS program said delays can occur when patients do not inform the CHS program of the alternate resources available to them, necessitating the CHS program doing the research itself.

Program officials also reported some delays related to the other three aspects of the process for determining eligibility for CHS payment. For example, officials from one CHS program said determining whether a patient is a member of a federally recognized tribe can result in a delay if they have never seen the patient before, and must obtain documentation of that patient's tribal affiliation. Similarly, officials from one CHS program said determining whether a patient resides in its CHSDA can result in a delay when the program needs to wait on documentation from patients confirming their addresses. Finally, one local CHS program reported that determining whether the program has been notified within required timeframes can result in a delay when an incorrect decision is made to deny the service, which is later overturned.

The complexity of determining whether services delivered to American Indians and Alaska Natives are eligible for CHS funding can also result in misunderstandings in which providers think payments have been delayed, when in fact the services provided were not eligible for payment. For example, IHS officials told us that sometimes patients do not understand CHS rules and seek emergency care from external providers, expecting the CHS program to cover it, when they are in fact not eligible for CHS. The officials also said that providers will send claims to the CHS program, assuming the patient and service are eligible, and expect to be paid. IHS does not issue eligibility cards to beneficiaries that would indicate to external providers their eligibility for CHS services or information about which local CHS program is responsible for payment. In a previous GAO review of the CHS program, several

58 United States Government Accountability Office

providers noted that, in the absence of a process they can use prior to providing service to determine patient eligibility for the CHS program, they submit claims for payment to the CHS program for all patients who self-identify as American Indian or Alaska Native or as eligible for the CHS program.[29] IHS officials said that they believe situations such as these—in which the provider will never be paid because the patient or service was not eligible, as opposed to situations in which the service is eligible but the payment process is prolonged—accounted for the majority of provider complaints about the timeliness of CHS payments.

Local CHS program officials noted that providers' lack of understanding of the complex CHS approval process was due in part to provider staff turnover or was exacerbated when the provider's billing functions were located out of state, which could result in delays in providing information needed to determine eligibility. These officials noted that education of provider staff was an ongoing necessity for CHS programs. Some IHS officials also noted that providing such training took staff time away from processing referrals. Officials from a number of CHS programs noted that they meet regularly with some of their high-volume providers to reconcile specific outstanding cases, and that over time these meetings have helped improve providers' understanding of the unique rules and procedures of the CHS program. However, officials also mentioned that turnover among provider staff often necessitated starting the process of educating providers again.

Complexities Associated with the CHS Processes for Paying Providers Also Can Affect Timeliness

Even after a service has been approved for CHS funding and a purchase order has been issued, delays can occur because of complexities in the last step in the payment process, which is managed by IHS's FI. Officials said this can occur because the providers do not understand the CHS process used by the FI. For example, officials said some providers do not understand that after receiving a purchase order, they also need to submit the claim to the FI to be paid.

Officials from local CHS programs and from the FI also reported examples where delays occurred because claims submitted by providers to the FI could not be matched to a corresponding purchase order in the FI's system. According to FI officials, it will issue only one payment for each purchase order. However, some purchase orders are intended to cover multiple services, such as for a series of physical therapy treatments. FI officials reported that providers sometimes submit claims for services that pertain to only a portion of the services authorized on the purchase order. In these cases, the FI pays for those services and closes out the purchase order. When providers submit subsequent claims related to other services that were authorized on the original purchase order, the FI is unable to pay the provider because the purchase order was closed. The provider then must go back to the CHS program to request a new purchase order and payment to the provider is delayed until the new purchase order is issued and submitted to the FI.

In addition to delays in payments to providers from issues matching claims and purchase orders, claims may be put on hold by the FI for other payment processing issues. One of the most common causes for claims being put on hold by the FI is when alternate resources have been confirmed, but the FI is waiting for information from the provider showing the amount paid by the other resources and the remaining amount that the provider is claiming from IHS.

CHS Staffing and Funding Availability Also Can Affect Timeliness of Payments to Providers

Local CHS program officials said insufficient CHS program staffing levels have affected their ability to issue timely purchase orders. IHS's staffing standards model established a staffing ratio based on the annual number of purchase orders authorized for health care services by a facility.[30] Some CHS program officials noted that their number of staff was below these standards. Further, local CHS program officials in programs that had a very small number of CHS staff (e.g., two or three) said that a vacancy or extended leave for even one staff person could affect the timeliness of issuing purchase orders—and one of these programs reported that related delays could be significant. Furthermore, IHS officials noted that, pursuant to agency practice, CHS funding has been used only to pay for services and not to increase staffing levels. As a result, recent increases in CHS funds have resulted in increased workloads, but staffing levels to manage the workloads have not increased. Staffing levels can affect the timeliness of payment for services, particularly for self-referrals where the entire process for determining eligibility for CHS payment does not begin until after the service is provided.

Officials from a few CHS programs also noted that funding issues could result in delays issuing a purchase order authorizing CHS funding, which

60 United States Government Accountability Office

would delay payments. In our prior work, some providers told us that delays in receiving payment from CHS of several months, or in some cases years, tended to occur when the CHS program's funding for the fiscal year had been depleted.[31] Again, as with other issues we have noted, funding shortages affect the amount of time it takes to pay providers for self-referrals more than IHS referrals because the self-referral service is already provided before the program determines if funds are available while for an IHS referral, the service can be postponed until funds become available.

Local CHS Program Practices for Implementing CHS Eligibility Regulations Vary, which May Contribute to Variations in Timeliness for Aspects of the Provider Payment Process

We found variation in local CHS program practices for implementing CHS eligibility rules, which may contribute to the variation in timeliness of the provider payment process across IHS areas. IHS officials said they allow flexibility in local CHS program practices because each has a different set of circumstances to consider. These circumstances include challenges regarding CHS funding levels among areas, state Medicaid program procedures for verifying eligibility, providers' familiarity with the CHS program, and the number of staff available to determine CHS eligibility for services.

During our interviews, IHS area and local CHS program officials reported differences in practices that could contribute to variation in the amount of time overall it takes to pay providers. Examples of these differences include:

Consideration of alternate resources. Local CHS programs varied in the actions they took while they were determining the extent of patients' alternate resources. One practice IHS area office officials said some local CHS program staff used, in certain circumstances, was to issue purchase orders to providers before patients' alternate resources were confirmed. In these cases, if the FI paid the claim before alternate resources were confirmed, the FI would seek to recover from the provider any overpayments for services covered by these alternate resources.

In contrast, some IHS area and local CHS program officials told us they do not issue purchase orders authorizing CHS payment for services until the availability of all possible alternate resources has been determined. Officials in one IHS area noted that they do this to preserve their limited CHS funds and provide access to care to as many patients as possible. Officials in this area reported that they were not able to fund all Priority 1 cases and that

Indian Health Service 61

issuing purchase orders and obligating CHS funds before alternate resources were confirmed could cause them to exhaust their CHS funds even earlier.

Requests for information from providers. Officials from some local CHS programs reported that they set time limits for providers to submit medical documents and deny CHS funding if providers do not submit the documents within that time. These limits ranged from a week to 45 days, and some of these programs automatically issued a denial if the medical documentation was not provided either at the same time the program was notified that services had been provided or by the specified time limit. CHS officials said these denials could be reconsidered if sufficient medical documentation were subsequently provided. In contrast, officials from another CHS program reported that it does not have established time limits within which providers must submit medical documentation.

Determination of medical priority. One practice that certain local CHS program officials reported was to make all decisions about the medical priority of requested services at their program's weekly medical committee meeting. In contrast, another reported practice was to have almost all medical priority determinations made by a clinician as soon as all necessary information is received. (Those determinations are subsequently reviewed by the committee.) A combination of both of these practices was also reported by another CHS program we spoke to, in which decisions on less complex cases were made by a clinician as soon as all necessary information was received, while determinations for more complicated cases waited until the next weekly medical committee meeting.

NEW COVERAGE OPTIONS IN PPACA MAY PROVIDE IHS AN OPPORTUNITY TO SIMPLIFY CHS ELIGIBILITY RULES

New health care coverage options available to many IHS beneficiaries as a result of provisions in PPACA could provide IHS with an opportunity to simplify the complex eligibility rules of the CHS program. IHS has stated that its overall service goal is to elevate the health status of American Indians and Alaska Natives to the highest possible level. However, as we and others have reported, limits on available resources have affected the services available to American Indians and Alaska Natives through the CHS program. For example, although funding for the CHS program significantly increased in recent years, IHS has reported that at current funding levels, most programs are approving only medically emergent referrals (Priority 1) and less urgent, routine or preventive care is deferred or denied pending additional appropriations. According to IHS, limits on available funding for the CHS program have caused the agency to establish its complex requirements for determining eligibility for CHS funds—including reliance on a medical priority rating system and limiting eligibility to individuals who reside in CHSDAs. These mechanisms are intended to enhance IHS's ability to stretch limited CHS dollars and extend services to more American Indians and Alaska Natives. As we previously reported, however, many American Indians and Alaska Natives may gain new health care coverage beginning in 2014 as a result of PPACA, which could alleviate some constraints on CHS program funds.[32]

If a better match is achieved between available funding and overall CHS program demand, IHS could have the opportunity to streamline eligibility requirements for the CHS program and to expand the services it pays for with CHS funds, assuming appropriation levels for the CHS program are maintained. Because the CHS program is generally the payer of last resort, if more American Indians and Alaska Natives gain new coverage, services that would have previously been paid for by the CHS program will be paid for by other payers. In addition, because some American Indians and Alaska Natives will have access to benefits packages through these other coverage options—benefits packages that may be more comprehensive than the IHS benefits available to them now—more may choose to obtain care outside of the IHS system entirely. This could help free up some CHS program funds, potentially creating a better match between available funding and overall program demand.

Some uncertainty remains, however, about the extent to which American Indians and Alaska Natives will obtain new health care coverage when PPACA is fully implemented. For example, not all states may choose to expand their Medicaid programs. In addition, we have reported previously on the challenges American Indians and Alaska Natives may face enrolling in Medicaid and other public insurance programs.[33] Some barriers are unique to the American Indian and Alaska Native population—such as individuals believing they should not have to apply for other public insurance programs because the federal government has a duty to provide them with health care as a result of treaties with Indian tribes. In our prior work, we recommended that IHS increase its direct outreach to American Indians and Alaska Natives who may be eligible for new coverage options to help ensure significant new enrollment in these options.[34]

Conclusion

The current CHS program's eligibility requirements reflect the method that IHS has chosen to stretch its funding to ensure that the most critical health services can be provided to the maximum number of beneficiaries. However, determining eligibility for CHS funding—including the need to ascertain each time a referral is received whether the patient met residency requirements and the service met medical priorities—is inherently complex. As currently structured, it is highly unlikely that the CHS program will be as quick a payer as some other payers because of the cumbersome steps involved in determining eligibility for each service.

PPACA will expand existing sources of health coverage and create new ones for American Indians and Alaska Natives, and this could affect the CHS program in a number of ways. In particular, if these changes significantly reduce the demand placed on CHS program funds, IHS may have the opportunity to not only pay for a greater range of services but also restructure the CHS program to include less stringent eligibility requirements. For example, increased availability of CHS funding due to increased access among American Indians and Alaska Natives to other sources of health care coverage options under PPACA could give IHS the opportunity to establish a set of defined benefits for IHS beneficiaries, which would alleviate the need for CHS programs and providers to carry out time-consuming medical priority determinations. The opportunity also may arise for IHS to make other changes, such as issuing a form of eligibility card to CHS-eligible patients to help providers understand when to send claims to IHS, and to which local CHS program a claim should be sent, helping improve the timeliness of provider payments.

In the interim, while the changes from PPACA are taking effect, IHS has the opportunity to continue to make improvements to the CHS program, including how it assesses the timeliness of provider payments and how it aligns CHS program staffing levels with workloads, and to proactively consider ways to streamline CHS eligibility requirements.

Recommendations for Executive Action

In an effort to ensure that IHS has meaningful information on the timeliness with which it issues purchase orders authorizing payment under the

64 United States Government Accountability Office

CHS program and to improve the timeliness of payments to providers, we recommend that the Secretary of HHS direct the Director of IHS to:

- modify IHS's claims data system to separately track IHS referrals and self-referrals, revise the GPRA measure for the CHS program so that it distinguishes between these two types of referrals, and establish separate timeframe targets for these referral types; and
- improve the alignment between CHS staffing levels and workloads by revising its current practices, where appropriate, to allow available funds to be used to pay for CHS program staff.

In addition, as HHS and IHS monitor the effect that new coverage options available to IHS beneficiaries through PPACA have on CHS program funds, we recommend that the Secretary of HHS direct the Director of IHS to proactively develop potential options to streamline program eligibility requirements.

AGENCY COMMENTS AND OUR EVALUATION

We provided a draft of this report to HHS for review and received written comments. In its comments, HHS concurred with two of our recommendations and did not concur with one recommendation.

HHS concurred with our recommendation that IHS modify its claims data system to separately track IHS referrals and self-referrals, revise the GPRA measure for the CHS program so that it distinguishes between these two types of referrals, and establish separate timeframe targets for these referral types. HHS also concurred with our recommendation that as HHS and IHS monitor the effect that new coverage options available to IHS beneficiaries through PPACA have on CHS program funds, IHS proactively develop potential options to streamline program eligibility requirements. HHS agreed with the premise that Medicaid eligibility expansion and private insurance for more American Indians and Alaska Natives will reduce the demand for CHS services and noted that IHS will monitor the effects of new coverage on program funds and develop options to improve and streamline the CHS program processes.

HHS did not concur with our recommendation that IHS improve the alignment between CHS staffing levels and workloads by revising its current practices, where appropriate, to allow available funds to be used to pay for

CHS program staff. In its response, HHS stated its intent to continue to only use CHS appropriations to purchase health care services and not to fund program staff, noting that available CHS program funds have not been sufficient to pay for all services and that at some facilities, funding was only sufficient to cover cases with the highest medical priority. We acknowledge the difficult challenges and choices faced by CHS programs when program funds are not sufficient to pay for all needed services. However, IHS has noted the importance of the agency maintaining an adequate workforce and has established staffing standards for the CHS program. As we reported, some IHS officials noted that their number of staff was below the staffing ratio established in IHS's staffing standards model, and local CHS program officials told us that insufficient CHS program staffing levels have affected their ability to issue timely purchase orders. Further, recent increases in CHS funding for services have resulted in increased workloads, while staffing levels to manage the workloads have not increased. For these reasons, we continue to believe that IHS should improve the alignment between CHS staffing levels and workloads, making use of all available funding, including CHS program funds, when appropriate, to do so.

Kathleen M. King
Director, Health Care

End Notes

[1] IHS defines an Indian tribe as any Indian tribe, band, nation, group, Pueblo, or community, including any Alaska Native village or Native group, which is federally recognized as eligible for the programs and services provided by the United States to Indians because of their status as Indians. 42 C.F.R. § 136.21(g)(2012).

[2] Under the Indian Self-Determination and Education Assistance Act, as amended, federally recognized Indian tribes can enter into self-determination contracts or self-governance compacts with the Secretary of Health and Human Services to take over the administration of IHS programs for Indians previously administered by IHS on their behalf. Self-governance compacts allow tribes to consolidate and assume administration of all programs, services, activities, and competitive grants administered throughout IHS, or portions thereof, that are carried out for the benefit of Indians because of their status as Indians. In contrast, self-determination contracts allow tribes to assume administration of a program, programs, or portions thereof. See 25 U.S.C. §§ 450f(a) (self-determination contracts) and 458aaa-4(b)(1) (self-governance compacts).

[3] IHS's 12 areas are: Aberdeen, Alaska, Albuquerque, Bemidji, Billings, California, Nashville, Navajo, Oklahoma City, Phoenix, Portland, and Tucson. All areas but Alaska and California include IHS-operated facilities.

66 United States Government Accountability Office

[4] Of the 243 local CHS programs, 66 are affiliated with IHS-operated facilities. The remaining 177 CHS programs are affiliated with tribally operated facilities.

[5] GAO, *Indian Health Service: Most American Indians and Alaska Natives Potentially Eligible for Expanded Health Coverage, but Action Needed to Increase Enrollment,* GAO-13-553 (Washington, D.C.: Sept. 5, 2013); *Indian Health Service: Capping Payment Rates for Nonhospital Services Could Save Millions of Dollars for Contract Health Services,* GAO-13-272 (Washington, D.C.: Apr. 11, 2013); *Indian Health Service: Action Needed to Ensure Equitable Allocation of Resources for the Contract Health Service Program,* GAO-12-446 (Washington, D.C.: Jun. 15, 2012); and *Indian Health Service: Increased Oversight Needed to Ensure Accuracy of Data Used for Estimating Contract Health Service Need,* GAO-11-767 (Washington, D.C.: Sept. 23, 2011).

[6] GAO-11-767 and GAO-13-272.

[7] GAO-11-767.

[8] GAO-13-553.

[9] Pub. L. No. 111-148, 124 Stat. 119, as amended by the Health Care and Education Reconciliation Act of 2010, Pub. L. No. 111-152, 124 Stat. 1029. For the purposes of this report, references to PPACA include the amendments made by the Health Care and Education Reconciliation Act of 2010.

[10] See Pub. L. No. 111-148, § 10221, 124 Stat. 119, 935 (2010) (enacting S. 1790, as reported by the Committee on Indian Affairs in the Senate in December 2009, into law with amendments); S. 1790, 111th Cong. §§ 137, 199 (2009).

[11] We did not obtain data on CHS claims that were authorized by tribally operated facilities, which account for approximately 54 percent of total CHS program payments. This review focused entirely on data and activities of CHS programs affiliated with IHS-operated facilities. These programs are located in 10 of the 12 IHS areas.

[12] GAO-13-553.

[13] IHS received about $800 million for the CHS program for fiscal year 2013.

[14] Eligibility requirements for CHS are in addition to meeting the requirements for direct care services.

[15] Tribal groups or IHS may submit requests to re-designate a CHSDA. These requests are reviewed by IHS and are subject to public comment.

[16] Medicaid is a jointly funded federal-state health care program that covers certain low-income individuals and families. Medicare is the federal government's health care insurance program for individuals aged 65 and older and for individuals with certain disabilities or end-stage renal disease.

[17] See 25 U.S.C. §§ 1621e, 1623; 42 C.F.R. § 136.61 (2012). There are certain exemptions to the CHS program's designation as a payer of last resort. For example, certain tribally funded health insurance plans are not considered alternate resources and the CHS program must pay for care before billing the tribally funded insurance plan. The CHS program must also pay for care provided to eligible American Indians and Alaska Natives before the crime victim compensation program, a federal program that provides compensation to victims of criminal violence.

[18] Tribal CHS programs must use medical priorities when making funding decisions but, unlike CHS programs affiliated with IHS-operated facilities, tribal programs may develop systems that differ from the set of priorities established by IHS.

[19] GAO, *Indian Health Service: Health Care Services Are Not Always Available to Native Americans,* GAO-05-789 (Washington, D.C.: Aug. 31, 2005); and GAO-11-767.

Indian Health Service
67

[20] PPACA established 133 percent of the federal poverty level as the income limit for expanded Medicaid eligibility; however, it also specifies that an individual's income be reduced by an amount equivalent to 5 percent of federal poverty level when determining Medicaid eligibility, which effectively raises the eligibility limit for newly eligible Medicaid recipients to 138 percent of the federal poverty level. See Pub. L. No. 111-148, §§ 2001(a)(1), 2002, 124 Stat., 271, 279; Pub. L. No. 111-152, § 1004(e), 124 Stat. 1036 (codified at 42 U.S.C. § 1396a(a)(10)(A)(i)(VIII) and 42 U.S.C. § 1396a(e)(14)(B)(I)).

[21] PPACA directed states to establish state-based exchanges by January 1, 2014. In states electing not to establish and operate such an exchange, PPACA requires the federal government to establish and operate such an exchange in the state. Pub. L. No. 111-148 §§ 1311(b)(1), 1321(c), 124. Stat., 173, 186 (codified at 42 U.S.C. §§ 18031(b) and 18041(c).

[22] PPACA provides for a federal premium tax credit for eligible individuals obtaining insurance through an exchange with incomes equal to or exceeding 100 and up to 400 percent of the federal poverty level, and who do not have access to public insurance, such as Medicaid. See Pub. L. No. 111-148, §§ 1401, 10105(a) – (c), 10108(h), 124 Stat. 213, 906, 914 ; Pub. L. No. 111-152, §§ 1001, 1004, 124 Stat. 1030, 1034(codified at 26 U.S.C. § 36B); 26 C.F.R. § 1.36B-2(a)(2013). In addition, American Indians and Alaska Natives who obtain insurance through an exchange are eligible for exemptions from cost-sharing, such as deductibles and copays, if they are members of federally recognized tribes and have a household income of not more than 300 percent of the federal poverty level or if the services are provided by Indian Health providers, regardless of the enrollee's income. See Pub. L. No. 111-148, § 1402(d), 124 Stat. 222 (codified at 42 U.S.C. § 18071(d)).

[23] Pub. L. No. 111-148, §§ 1331, 10104(o), 124 Stat. 199, 902 (codified at 42 U.S.C. § 18051).

[24] GAO-13-553.

[25] IHS does not have a performance measure for the second step of the payment process—the time between the date the purchase order is issued and the date IHS's FI receives the claim from the provider seeking payment. IHS has little involvement in this step of the payment process. During this period, the provider submits the claim to the FI; IHS has not established a deadline for the provider to do this.

[26] GAO, *Executive Guide: Effectively Implementing the Government Performance and Results Act,* GAO/GGD-96-118, (Washington D.C.: June 1996); and *Agencies' Strategic Plans Under GPRA: Key Questions to Facilitate Congressional Review,* GAO/GGD-10.1.16 (Washington D.C.: May 1997).

[27] See 25 U.S.C. § 1621s.

[28] Our analysis showed that 83 percent of claims were paid by the FI within 1 month of receiving the provider's claim. This difference between our analysis and the FI reports may be explained by the fact that our analysis included claims that were at one time not clean.

[29] GAO-11-767.

[30] According to the model, each facility that issues 50 or more purchase orders should have a CHS Manager staff and one CHS staff position for every 700 purchase orders issued annually. Plus, the facility should have a data entry clerk if the CHS program uses the automated system for referrals.

[31] GAO-11-767.

[32] GAO-13-553.

[33] See GAO, *Medicare and Medicaid: CMS and State Efforts to Interact with the Indian Health Service and Indian Tribes,* GAO-08-724 (Washington, D.C.: Jul. 11, 2008).

[34] GAO-13-533.

In: The Indian Health Service
Editor: Pamela M. Agnelli

ISBN: 978-1-63321-582-5
© 2014 Nova Science Publishers, Inc.

Chapter 3

INDIAN HEALTH CARE: IMPACT OF THE AFFORDABLE CARE ACT (ACA)[*]

Elayne J. Heisler

SUMMARY

On March 23, 2010, President Obama signed into law a comprehensive health care reform bill, the Patient Protection and Affordable Care Act (ACA; P.L. 111-148). The law, among other things, reauthorizes the Indian Health Care Improvement Act (P.L. 94-437, IHCIA), which authorizes many programs and services provided by the Indian Health Service (IHS). In addition, it makes several changes that may affect American Indians and Alaska Natives enrolled in and receiving services from the Medicare, Medicaid, and State Children's Health Insurance Program (CHIP)—also called Social Security Act (SSA) health benefit programs. The ACA also includes changes to private health insurance that may affect American Indians and Alaska Natives and may affect tribes that offer private health insurance.

IHCIA authorizes many IHS programs and services, sets out the national policy for health services administered to Indians, and articulates the federal goal of ensuring the highest possible health status for Indians, including urban Indians. In addition, it authorizes direct collections from Medicare, Medicaid, and other third-party insurers. Prior to the ACA,

---

[*] This is an edited, reformatted and augmented version of a Congressional Research Service publication R41152, prepared for Members and Committees of Congress, dated January 9, 2014.

IHCIA was last reauthorized in FY2000, although programs continued to receive appropriations in later years. The ACA reauthorizes IHCIA and extends authorizations of appropriations for IHCIA programs indefinitely. It amends a number of sections of IHCIA in general, to permit tribal organizations (TOs) and urban Indian organizations (UIOs) to apply for contract and grant programs for which they were not previously eligible; to create new mental health prevention and treatment programs; and to require demonstration projects to construct modular and mobile health facilities in order to expand health services available through IHS, Indian Tribes (ITs), and TOs. It also made several organizational changes to IHS. It requires IHS to establish an Office of Direct Service Tribes to serve tribes that receive their health care and other services directly from IHS as opposed to receiving services through IHS-funded facilities or programs operated by ITs or TOs. In addition, the law requires IHS to develop a plan to establish a new area office to serve tribes in Nevada and requires the Secretary of the Department of Health and Human Services (HHS) to appoint a new IHS Director of HIV/AIDS Prevention and Treatment.

In addition to reauthorizing IHCIA, the ACA includes a number of provisions that may affect American Indians and Alaska Natives who have private insurance coverage or who receive services through SSA health benefit programs. With regard to private insurance coverage, the ACA provides a special enrollment period for American Indians and Alaska Natives who may enroll in private insurance offered through an exchange and exempts certain American Indians and Alaska Natives from the requirement to obtain insurance coverage. Under regulation, additional American Indians and Alaska Natives may also be exempt from the ACA requirement to obtain insurance coverage. With regard to SSA health benefit programs, the new law permits specified Indian entities to determine Medicaid and CHIP eligibility and extends the period during which IHS, IT, and TO services are reimbursed for all Medicare Part B services, indefinitely, beginning January 1, 2010. Prior to the ACA, authority for these facilities to receive Medicare Part B reimbursements for certain specified services had expired on January 1, 2010.

INTRODUCTION

On March 23, 2010, President Obama signed into law a comprehensive health care reform bill, the Patient Protection and Affordable Care Act (ACA),[1] which, among other things, reauthorizes the Indian Health Care Improvement Act (IHCIA[2]).[3] This report, one of a series of CRS products on the ACA, summarizes some of the key changes made in the reauthorization of

Indian Health Care: Impact of the Affordable Care Act (ACA)   71

IHCIA. In addition, the report summarizes other ACA provisions related to American Indians and Alaska Natives enrolled in and receiving services from Medicare, Medicaid, and the State Children's Health Insurance Program (CHIP)—also called SSA health benefit programs.[4] It also discusses ACA changes to private health insurance coverage that may affect American Indians' and Alaska Natives' access to private health insurance coverage.

The report begins with an overview of the Indian Health Service (IHS) and IHCIA. It then discusses each of the eight titles in IHCIA and how the ACA amends each of these titles. Finally, the report discusses other ACA changes that may affect American Indians and Alaska Natives. For each topic, including each IHCIA title, discussed, the report first gives a brief description for context, and then describes the changes made by the ACA.

This report is primarily for reference purposes. The material in it is intended to provide context to help the reader better understand the intent of ACA's reauthorization of IHCIA at the time of enactment. In general, this report does not track ongoing ACA-related regulatory and other implementation activities.

OVERVIEW OF INDIAN HEALTH CARE

The Indian Health Service (IHS), an agency within the Department of Health and Human Services (HHS), provides health care for approximately 2.2 million eligible American Indians/Alaska Natives through a system of programs and facilities located on or near Indian reservations, and through contractors in certain urban areas.[5] IHS provides services in 35 states, subdivided into 12 geographic "Areas" that consist of one or more states.[6] Each Area is administered by an Area Office; Areas, in turn, are further subdivided into service units that consist of one or more facilities. IHS may provide services directly, or Indian tribes (ITs) or tribal organizations (TOs) may operate IHS facilities and programs themselves through self-determination contracts and self-governance compacts negotiated with IHS.[7] Although most IHS facilities are located on or near reservations, IHS also funds urban Indian health projects (UIHPs), through grants or contracts to urban Indian organizations (UIOs).

The IHS provides an array of medical services, including inpatient, ambulatory, emergency, dental, public health nursing, and preventive health care.[8] The IHS does not have a defined medical benefit package that excludes or includes specific conditions or types of health care. Besides providing general clinical health services, the IHS also focuses on health conditions prevalent among American Indians and Alaska Natives such as infant mortality, diabetes, and hepatitis B. In addition, IHS provides mental health and alcohol and substance abuse services because, compared to the overall U.S. population, American Indians and Alaska Natives are more likely to die from alcoholism-related diseases or to commit suicide.[9]

In addition to health services, the IHS funds projects related to health care facilities and sanitation. Specifically, the IHS funds the construction, equipping, and maintenance of hospitals, health centers, clinics, and other health care delivery facilities, both those operated by the IHS and those operated by tribes. In order to improve the health of, and reduce the incidence of disease among, American Indians and Alaska Natives, the IHS also funds the construction of water supply and sewage facilities and solid waste disposal systems, and provides technical assistance for the operation and maintenance of such facilities. The IHS has attributed decreases in gastrointestinal disease among American Indians and Alaska Natives to improved sanitation facilities.[10]

INDIAN HEALTH CARE IMPROVEMENT ACT

The Indian Health Care Improvement Act, as passed in 1976 and subsequently amended, authorized many specific IHS activities,[11] set out the national policy for health services administered to Indians, and declared that it was a federal goal to improve the health status and conditions of the IHS service population. IHCIA also authorized direct collections from Medicare, Medicaid, and other third-party insurers for American Indians and Alaska Natives receiving services at facilities operated by the IHS, an IT, or a TO. IHCIA gave IHS authority to grant funding to UIOs to provide health care services to urban Indians, and established substance abuse treatment programs, Indian health professions recruitment programs, and many other programs. Prior to the ACA, IHCIA was last fully reauthorized by the Indian Health Amendments of 1992,[12] which extended authorizations of its appropriations through FY2000. In 2000, all IHCIA authorizations of appropriations were extended through FY2001.[13] Prior to reauthorizing IHCIA in the ACA, lawmakers introduced multiple reauthorization bills.[14] Despite the lapse in authorization of appropriations during this period, Congress continued to appropriate funds for IHCIA programs.[15]

IHCIA Reauthorization in the ACA

ACA Title X, "Strengthening Quality, Affordable Health Care for All Americans," in Subtitle B, "Provisions Relating to Title II," Part III, amends and enacts the "Indian Health Care Improvement Reauthorization and Extension Act of 2009 (S. 1790)," as reported by the Senate Committee on Indian Affairs on December 16, 2009.[16] Title II, "Role of Public Programs," Subtitle K, "Protections for American Indians and Alaska Natives," contains provisions related to American Indians and Alaska Natives in SSA health benefit programs and in the private health insurance exchange established by the ACA.[17] In addition, other sections of the ACA include changes related to private insurance that may affect American Indians and Alaska Natives. The ACA reauthorizes IHCIA permanently and indefinitely; it appropriates such sums as may be necessary for FY2010 and each fiscal year thereafter, to remain available until expended. The ACA maintains IHCIA's eight titles but amends and adds a number of sections to each of the titles. *Table 1* summarizes the changes that the ACA makes to IHCIA.

Table 1. IHCIA Reauthorization Summary

IHCIA Title Name and Subject	ACA
Title I-Indian Health Manpower Authorizes workforce programs to increase the supply of providers at IHS facilities	Maintains title's major sections; repeals section authorizing appropriations for the title; expands use of community health aide workers at IHS-funded facilities; adds a new section funding a demonstration to address IHS health professional shortages; and exempts employees at IHS-funded facilities from certain licensing, registration requirements and related fees.
Title II-Health Services Authorizes IHS health services, research, payments for service-related transportation, payment for services provided through contracts with outside providers (i.e., Contract Health Services [CHS])[a]	Maintains title's major sections; repeals section authorizing appropriations for the title; amends authorization for two funds (Indian Health Care Improvement Fund and Catastrophic Health Emergency Fund); expands IHS authority for diabetes, cancer screening, and long-term care programs; and amends sections related to the CHS program.
Title III-Health Facilities Authorizes construction and renovation of IHS facilities; sets procedures by which construction and renovation projects are selected	Maintains title's major sections; repeals section authorizing appropriations for the title; amends IHS construction priority system; and adds new sections requiring grants to build modular and mobile facilities.

Table 1. (Continued)

IHCIA Title Name and Subject	ACA
Title IV-Access to Health Services Authorizes IHS programs to bill Medicare, Medicaid, and private insurance	Maintains title's major sections; repeals section authorizing appropriations for the title; adds the State Children's Health Insurance Program to programs that IHS is authorized to bill; adds new sections permitting ITs, TOs, and UIOs to purchase federal employee health and life insurance benefits for their employees; expands IHS collaboration with the Department of Veterans Affairs and the Department of Defense.
Title V-Health Services for Urban Indians Authorizes grants to UIOs for health projects to serve urban Indians	Maintains title's major sections; repeals section authorizing appropriations for the title; expands grant opportunities available t UIOs.
Title VI-Organization Improvements Establishes IHS's organizational position within HHS; the position of Director of IHS; and requires an automated management information system for IHS record-keeping	Maintains title's major sections; establishes that the IHS Director should report directly to the HHS Secretary; adds new sections requiring (1) an Office of Direct Service Tribes; and (2) a plan to create a new Nevada Area Office.
Title VII-Behavioral Health Programs Authorizes programs related to behavioral health prevention and treatment	Replaces IHCIA Title VII with new language authorizing new comprehensive behavioral health and treatment programs. Includes a new subsection authorizing programs related to youth suicide prevention.
Title VIII-Miscellaneous Requires the IHS Director to submit a number of reports; establishes IHS eligibility for health services; and defines California Indians, amongst other provisions	Maintains title's major sections; repeals section authorizing appropriations for the title; adds new sections that, among other things, establish (1) a prescription drugs monitoring program; (2) an IHS Director of HIV/AIDS Prevention and Treatment; and (3) new requirements for the IHS budget requests to reflect inflation and changes in the IHS service population.

Source: CRS analysis of P.L. 94-437, as amended (IHCIA), and P.L. 111-148 (ACA).

[a] Beginning with the FY2014 budget justification, this program is now referred to as the purchased/referred care program. See U.S. Dept. of Health and Human Services, Indian Health Service, Fiscal Year 2014 Indian Health Service Justification of Estimates, http://www.ihs.gov/BudgetFormulation/documents/FY2014BudgetJustification.pdf.

Definitions[18]

The ACA defines a number of new Indian-related terms. Two of the new terms most frequently used are Indian Health Program and Tribal Health Program. "Indian Health Program" (IHP) is defined as (1) any health program administered by the IHS, (2) any Tribal Health Program, or (3) any Indian tribe or tribal organization to which the Secretary provides funding under the Buy Indian Act.[19] "Tribal Health Program" (THP) is defined as any IT or TO operating any health program, service, function, activity, or facility funded, in whole or part, by the IHS through, or provided for in, a contract or compact with the IHS under the Indian Self-Determination and Education Assistance Act (ISDEAA).[20] In addition, the bill maintains a number of IHCIA-defined terms.

SELECTED MAJOR CHANGES TO IHCIA IN THE ACA

Purposes and Findings: Adds a new finding that articulates that it is a major national goal of the United States to provide resources, processes, and structure that will enable ITs and tribal members to obtain the quantity and quality of health care services and opportunities that will eradicate health disparities between Indians and the general population.

Appropriations: Consolidates authorizations of appropriations into a single provision, authorizes such sums as may be necessary, and extends authorizations of appropriations indefinitely. In addition, the ACA repeals the separate authorizations of appropriations that had been included at the end of each IHCIA title or had been included in specific IHCIA sections.

Expanded Access to UIOs and TOs: Permits TOs and UIOs to apply for grant and contract programs for which these entities were previously not eligible.

Behavioral Health Programs: Expands mental health services to create a comprehensive behavioral health and treatment program. It includes programs related to youth suicide prevention and increases IT and TO access to grants sponsored by the Substance Abuse and Mental Health Services Administration (SAMHSA).[21]

Payor of Last Resort: States that IHS is the payor of last resort for all services provided. Prior to the ACA,[22] IHS was the payor of last resort only for contract health services (CHS)—services that IHS, ITs, or TOs may purchase, through contracts, from private providers in instances where the IHP cannot provide the needed care.[23]

Indians in SSA Programs: Extends Medicare payments to hospitals operated by IHS, ITs, or TOs, and permits Indian entities to determine Medicaid and CHIP eligibility in order to facilitate American Indian and Alaska Native enrollment in Medicaid and CHIP.

Office of Direct Service Tribes: Requires that IHS establish an Office of Direct Service Tribes to serve tribes that receive their health care and other services directly from IHS rather than through facilities or programs operated by ITs or TOs.

Nevada Area Office: Requires a plan to establish a new area office to serve tribes in Nevada.

Demonstration Projects: Includes two facilities demonstration projects that will award funds for IHS, ITs, or TOs to construct modular and mobile health facilities.

IHCIA TITLE I: INDIAN HEALTH, HUMAN RESOURCES, AND DEVELOPMENT

IHCIA Title I included provisions related to increasing the number of American Indians and Alaska Natives entering the health professions in order to increase the supply of health professionals available to facilities and programs operated by IHS, ITs, and TOs. At the time of the ACA's enactment, the IHS had high vacancy rates in many of its health professions—over 20% for physicians, and over 15% for dentists and nurses, for instance, as of January 2010.[24] IHCIA authorized a number of workforce programs, including, for example, scholarship and loan repayment programs, to encourage health professionals to work at facilities operated by the IHS or ITs; funding for continuing education for IHS employees; funding for advanced training and for recruitment and retention for individuals working at facilities operated by the IHS, an IT, a TO, or a UIO; training for nursing; and programs to encourage American Indians and Alaska Natives to enter medicine. In addition, Title I authorized two innovative health professions programs: the community health representative (CHR) program, which permits the training of American Indians and Alaska Natives to serve as paraprofessionals who provide health care, health promotion, and disease prevention services at IHS facilities; and the community health aide program (CHAP), which provides

Indian Health Care: Impact of the Affordable Care Act (ACA) 77

training for Alaska Natives to serve as health aides or community health practitioners.

The ACA maintains and reauthorizes a number of these health professions programs. It expands the CHAP program to areas outside of Alaska, but excludes CHAP's dental health aide therapist program in Alaska from states outside of Alaska unless an IT or a TO, in a state authorizing such a program, elects to include it. The ACA also includes additional requirements for the Secretary to facilitate the implementation of the CHAP dental health aide program by ITs and TOs and prohibits the Secretary from filling IHS program vacancies for certified dentists with dental health aide therapists.

IHCIA TITLE II: HEALTH SERVICES

IHCIA Title II authorized a number of specific health programs and activities, including mental health programs, prevention activities, diabetes and tuberculosis programs, Indian women's health, Indian school health education programs, epidemiological centers, and a fund for the elimination of backlogs and deficiencies among Indian health programs (called the Indian Health Care Improvement Fund (IHCIF)), and other programs. The title also included provisions relating to CHS delivery areas in several states.[25] CHS services are limited to American Indians and Alaska Natives living in defined geographic areas called CHS delivery areas.

The ACA reauthorizes the IHCIF as well as the Catastrophic Health Emergency Fund (which provides extra funding to facilities with extraordinary medical costs because of disasters and catastrophic illnesses). It expands the range of health promotion and disease prevention activities required to be provided, and includes new authorizations for hospice care, assisted living, longterm care, and home- and community-based services for disabled elderly persons. Title II also includes sections related to the Indians into Psychology Program, the Indian youth grant program, epidemiology centers, prevention and control of communicable and infectious diseases, requirements for prompt IHS payments to CHS providers, and timely notification to providers that CHS patients are exempt from payment for CHS services.

The ACA also requires the Secretary to maintain any existing or future model diabetes projects, and requires recurring funding for THPs' model diabetes projects.

IHCIA TITLE III: FACILITIES

IHCIA Title III includes provisions related to health care and sanitation facilities. IHS funds the construction, equipping, and maintenance of hospitals, health centers, clinics, and other health care delivery facilities for facilities operated by IHS and tribes. IHS also funds the construction of sanitation facilities, including water-supply and sewage facilities and solid waste disposal systems, and provides technical assistance for the operation and maintenance of such facilities. IHCIA required the Secretary to ensure that pay rates on such facility construction or renovation projects, if funded under IHCIA Title III, must not fall below the prevailing local wage rates, as determined in accordance with the Davis-Bacon Act.[26]

The ACA maintains current pay rate requirements; it requires the development of a priority system for construction of Indian health care facilities, with a methodology to be reported to Congress, and with priority lists for the 10 highest-priority facilities in five categories of facilities (inpatient, outpatient, specialized facilities, staff quarters, and facility-related hostels). The priority system also permits new facilities to be nominated at least every three years, but protects the priority of facilities at the top of the current lists for construction. The law also requires consultation with ITs and TOs to develop innovative approaches to solving unmet healthcare facility needs, and includes an "area distribution fund" as an option for such innovation. Under the concept of an area distribution fund, each IHS area would receive at least some health facilities construction funding, which was not the case prior to IHCIA's reauthorization.

The ACA creates a facilities needs assessment workgroup and a facilities appropriations advisory board in IHS. It maintains authorization for construction of sanitation and water-supply facilities, requires reports to Congress on the priority system for such facilities, authorizes the Secretary to accept major renovations or modernizations of Indian health facilities carried out by ITs, and requires grants to ITs and TOs for construction or upgrading of small ambulatory care facilities.

The ACA also includes a new provision that authorizes the Secretary to accept funding from any other source for facilities construction. It explicitly authorizes other federal agencies to transfer funds, equipment, or supplies to the Secretary for facilities construction and related activities, makes sanitation as well as health care facilities eligible, requires the Secretary to establish health and sanitation facility construction standards by regulation, and specifies that the Secretary's receipt of funds from other sources would not

Indian Health Care: Impact of the Affordable Care Act (ACA) 79

affect priorities established under Section 301 of IHCIA Title III. In addition, the ACA authorizes a new demonstration grant program for modular component health care facilities in Indian communities, and a new demonstration program for mobile health stations for providing specialty health care services.

IHCIA TITLE IV: ACCESS TO HEALTH SERVICES

IHCIA Title IV contained sections related to billing, and enrollment in, the Medicare and Medicaid programs operated by the Centers for Medicare & Medicaid Services (CMS);[27] a section authorizing appropriations; and a section that authorized emergency CHS services. The title's authorization for IHS health care facilities to receive reimbursements from the Medicare and Medicaid program was a major component of the original IHCIA passed in 1976. Prior to the ACA, IHCIA did not mention funds received under the State Children's Health Insurance (CHIP) program because the program was enacted after IHCIA was last reauthorized.[28]

Title IV contained provisions related to billing and receiving reimbursements from the Medicare and Medicaid programs. Specifically, IHCIA (1) authorized a demonstration project that permits ITs or TOs operating under ISDEAA contracts or compacts to directly bill CMS for Medicare and Medicaid payments; (2) required direct billing reimbursements be placed into a "special fund" that must be used first to achieve compliance with Medicare and Medicaid requirements and then, if excess funds exist, to improve health services available to the population the facility serves; (3) specified the auditing and other requirements related to direct billing; and (4) required that the federal government pay 100% of the cost of all Medicaid services billed.[29] In addition, IHCIA required that reimbursements from Medicare or Medicaid may not be considered when determining annual Indian health appropriations, required the Secretary to submit a report accounting for Medicare and Medicaid funds reimbursed to IHS, and required the Secretary to make grants to ITs or TOs to facilitate enrollment in Medicare and Medicaid.

The ACA maintains SSA health benefit reimbursement requirements, but adds reimbursements received from the CHIP program to these requirements. For example, reimbursements received from CHIP are included in the requirement that reimbursements from SSA health benefit programs not be taken into account when determining IHS appropriations. The ACA also expands and makes permanent the prior demonstration project that permitted

ITs or TOs operating under ISDEAA contracts or compacts to directly bill CMS for Medicare and Medicaid payments and excludes such direct billing reimbursements from the special fund. The ACA also includes grants for outreach and enrollment into SSA health benefit programs and maintains and expands current authorization to recover reimbursements from third-party entities and to credit such reimbursements to the facility that provided the services. In addition, the ACA authorizes ITs, TOs, and UIOs to use SSA health benefit funds and ISDEAA funds to purchase health care coverage and permits ITs, TOs, and UIOs to purchase Federal Employee Health Benefits and Federal Employee Group Life Insurance coverage for their employees. The ACA requires that federal health care programs accept an entity operated by the IHS, an IT, a TO, or a UIO as a provider eligible to receive payments, on the same basis as other qualified providers, if it meets the applicable licensure requirements for its provider type, regardless of whether the facility obtains the applicable license. The ACA also applies this licensing requirement to providers working at Indian entities, and prohibits providers and entities that are excluded from receiving reimbursements from other federal programs from receiving reimbursements from Indian entities.

The ACA expands IHS's relationship with the Department of Veterans Affairs (VA) and the Department of Defense (DOD) by authorizing increased coordination to treat Indian veterans.[30] In addition, the ACA requires the Secretary to conduct a study to determine the feasibility of treating the Navajo Nation as a state for Medicaid purposes, for Indians living within the Navajo Nation's boundaries.[31]

IHCIA TITLE V: HEALTH SERVICES FOR URBAN INDIANS

IHCIA Title V directed the HHS Secretary to make contracts with or grants to UIOs for health projects to serve urban Indians, and set requirements for the contracts and grants. Such grants or contracts are under the authority of the Snyder Act,[32] not the ISDEAA. The purpose of Title V programs is to make health services more accessible and available to urban Indians. Urban Indian Health Projects (UIHPs) may serve a wider range of eligible persons than the general IHS health care programs, including not only members of federally recognized tribes but also members of terminated[33] or state-recognized tribes, as well as their children and grandchildren.

Thirty-four UIHPs operate at 41 locations; they offer different programs with some offering different services, such as ambulatory health care, health promotion and education, immunizations, case management, child abuse prevention and treatment, and behavioral health services.[34] Besides IHS grants and contracts, UIHPs receive funding from state and private sources, patient fees,[35] Medicaid, Medicare, and other non-IHS federal programs.[36]

The ACA enables UIOs to expand their urban Indian health programs by permitting UIOs to establish a UIHP in urban centers other than where the UIO is located; prior to the ACA UIOs could only establish UIHPs in the urban area where the UIO was based. In addition, the ACA provides UIOs access to goods and services purchased through federal prime vendors, by deeming UIOs with Title V contracts or grants to be federal executive agencies under the section of the Federal Property and Administrative Services Act of 1974[37] concerning federal sources of supply. It also authorizes the Secretary to donate excess or surplus property to such UIOs and to permit the UIOs to use HHS facilities. The ACA also expands to UIOs the authorization for a number of programs currently only at IHS, IT, or TO facilities. For example, the ACA authorizes UIOs to employ Community Health Representatives (CHRs) trained under the CHR program authorized under current IHCIA Title I, and authorizes the Secretary to establish programs for UIOs that are identical to IHS programs for prevention of communicable diseases, for behavioral health prevention and treatment, and for youth multi-drug abuse prevention and treatment. The ACA also authorizes grants to UIOs for the development and implementation of health information technology, telemedicine, and related infrastructure.

IHCIA TITLE VI: ORGANIZATIONAL IMPROVEMENTS

IHCIA Title VI established IHS as part of the Public Health Service (PHS)[38] within HHS, and is administered by a Director who reports to the HHS Assistant Secretary for Health. IHCIA Title VI also required the Secretary to establish an automated management information system for IHS and IHPs, with a patient privacy component, and requires that patients have access to their own IHS records.

The ACA maintains the placement of IHS in PHS, but directs the head of IHS to report directly to the HHS Secretary. It also maintains requirements regarding the automated management information system. The ACA also adds two new requirements: the Secretary must establish an IHS Office of Direct

82 Elayne J. Heisler

Service Tribes (for tribes served directly by IHS instead of under ISDEAA), and the Secretary must submit to Congress a plan to create a new Nevada Area Office (Nevada is currently within the Phoenix Area Office).

IHCIA TITLE VII: BEHAVIORAL HEALTH PROGRAMS

IHCIA Title VII authorized alcohol and substance abuse programs, including grant and contract programs to provide comprehensive alcohol and substance abuse prevention and treatment services. It required coordination with the Department of the Interior to assess the need for such services and to provide community education in alcohol and substance abuse; requires services to specified groups including women and youth; and authorizes training and community education programs, demonstration projects to establish substance abuse counseling education curricula at tribally operated community colleges, and grants for preventing, treating, and diagnosing fetal alcohol syndrome (FAS) and fetal alcohol effects. In addition, Title VII included authorization for substance abuse treatment projects in specified locations in New Mexico, Arizona, and Alaska.

The ACA replaces current IHCIA Title VII with new language that authorizes programs to create a "comprehensive behavioral health prevention and treatment program" providing a "continuum of behavioral health care." For example, the ACA includes programs related to behavioral health prevention and treatment; provisions related to training and licensure requirements for the behavioral health workforce serving at facilities operated by IHS, ITs, or TOs; specific programs to treat Indian women and youth; and programs to treat and prevent child sexual abuse and fetal alcohol disorder. Many of these programs are similar to those that were authorized in IHCIA Title VII. The ACA also includes a new program to award grants to ITs and TOs to carry out demonstration projects using telehealth technology to provide youth suicide prevention and treatment services and authorizes appropriations of $1.5 million for each of FY2010-FY2013 for the new program. In addition, the ACA includes authorization for programs to prevent and treat domestic and sexual violence, and includes a number of requirements for the Secretary to facilitate ITs' and TOs' applying for, and inclusion in, grants from SAMHSA. It also requires the Secretary to carry out activities to increase the use of pre-doctoral psychology and psychiatry interns in order to increase access to mental health services, and authorizes the Secretary to establish a demonstration program through SAMSHA to test a culturally appropriate life

Indian Health Care: Impact of the Affordable Care Act (ACA) 83

skills curriculum to prevent suicide in American Indian and Alaska Native adolescents. The ACA also authorizes an appropriation of $1 million for each of FY2010-FY2014 for the Secretary to establish a grant program to award grants to ITs, TOs, or other entities to establish life skills curriculums to prevent suicide in schools located in high suicide areas that serve Indian children.

IHCIA TITLE VIII: MISCELLANEOUS

IHCIA Title VIII included a number of separate provisions covering reports, regulations, an IHCIA implementation plan, abortion, eligibility for IHS services, service unit funding reductions, and a variety of other topics.

The ACA maintains a number of IHCIA requirements including those requiring reports, regulations, an IHCIA implementation plan, and those defining individuals eligible for IHS services. The ACA extends the prior IHCIA limitation on the use of federal funds for abortions to IHS, and applies restrictions contained in other federal laws to IHS appropriations. The ACA also makes IHP and UIO medical quality assurance records confidential, and adds several new required reports. The ACA requires a new report on disease and injury prevention, and two new Government Accountability Office reports: (1) on the coordination of Indian health care services provided through IHS, Medicare, Medicaid, or CHIP, or with tribal, state, or local funds;[39] and (2) on the CHS program, including CHS payments to providers (since CHS providers still experience late payments).[40] The ACA also requires that IHS budget requests reflect inflation and changes in the IHS service population, and requires the establishment of a prescription drug monitoring program at IHP and UIO facilities. The ACA also permits a tribe operating an IHS health program through an ISDEAA self-governance compact to charge Indians for services; adds language stating that the United States has no liability for injury or death resulting from traditional health care practices; and establishes an IHS Director of HIV/AIDS Prevention and Treatment.

NATIVE HAWAIIAN HEALTH CARE REAUTHORIZATION

The ACA also includes the reauthorization of the Native Hawaiian Health Care Act of 1988,[41] which authorizes health education, health promotion, disease prevention services, and health professions scholarship programs for Native Hawaiians.[42] It extends the act's authorizations of appropriations through FY2019, permits a specified school in Hawaii to offer educational programs to Native Hawaiians first, and amends a definition in the act.[43]

ACA PRIVATE HEALTH INSURANCE CHANGES

The ACA makes significant changes to private health insurance coverage that may affect certain American Indians and Alaska Natives. The ACA includes a requirement for individuals, with certain exceptions, to obtain health insurance or be subject to a financial penalty (i.e., the individual mandate). It also establishes health insurance exchanges to provide individuals and small employers access to purchase private health insurance plans.[44] With respect to benefits and penalties, these provisions use several different statutory definitions of "Indian"; however, these definitions define the same groups as "Indian" (see text box for definitions and their uses). The following definitions of "Indian" and "Indian Tribe" are used for these ACA sections:

- Section 1311(c)(6)(d) requires a special enrollment period for American Indians and Alaska Natives, as defined in IHCIA, who are seeking to enroll in private health insurance plans offered through the health insurance exchanges. This special enrollment period permits members of federally recognized Indian Tribes to enroll in a qualified health plan monthly and to change their plan monthly.[45] In general, individuals who enroll in a qualified health plan through an exchange may only do so during a defined period and may only change plans annually.[46]
- Section 1501 exempts members of Indian tribes (as defined in the Internal Revenue Code [IRC]) from any penalty associated with a failure to comply with the individual mandate.[47]
- Section 1411(b)(5)(A) requires an "Indian" (not defined) who is seeking an exemption from the individual mandate to provide the Secretary of HHS with certain documentation that demonstrates his or her eligibility for this exemption.
- Section 1402(d) exempts American Indians and Alaska Natives who meet the definition of "Indian" in ISDEAA and whose income is not more than 300% of the federal poverty level from cost-sharing

Indian Health Care: Impact of the Affordable Care Act (ACA)   85

requirements if they are enrolled in a private health insurance plan offered through the exchange.

- Section 9021 uses the IRC definition of Indian to exclude the value of Indian tribe health benefits from calculations of gross income for tax purposes.[48]

The Three Definitions of Indian and Indian Tribe in the ACA

Indian Health Care Improvement Act (IHCIA) definition: IHCIA defines "Indian(s)" as "any person who is a member of an Indian tribe. IHCIA defines the term "Indian tribe" to mean "...any Indian tribe, band, nation, or other organized group or community, including any Alaska Native village or group or regional or village corporation as defined in or established pursuant to the Alaska Native Claims Settlement Act (85 Stat. 688), which is recognized as eligible for the special programs and services provided by the United States to Indians because of their status as Indians." ACA Usage: All of the IHCIA reauthorization (Title X) and Section 1311, which established a special enrollment period for Indians to enroll in private health insurance plans offered through the exchange.

Indian Self Determination and Education Assistance Act (ISDEAA) definition: ISDEAA defines an "Indian" "as a person who is a member of an Indian tribe." ISDEAA defines "Indian tribes" as "...any Indian tribe, band, nation, or other organized group or community, including any Alaska Native village or regional or village corporation as defined in or established pursuant to the Alaska Native Claims Settlement Act (85 Stat. 688) [43 U.S.C. § §1601 et seq.], which is recognized as eligible for the special programs and services provided by the United States to Indians because of their status as Indians." ACA Usage: Exempts Indians from cost sharing if they are enrolled in a plan offered through the private health insurance exchange.

Internal Revenue Code (IRC) definition: The term "Indian tribe" means any Indian tribe, band, nation, pueblo, or other organized group or community, including any Alaska Native village, or regional or village corporation, as defined in, or established pursuant to, the Alaska Native Claims Settlement Act (43 U.S.C. § §1601 et seq.) which is recognized as eligible for the special programs and services provided by the United States to Indians because of their status as Indians.

> ACA Usage: Exempts Indians from penalties associated with the failure to comply with the requirement to have health insurance coverage (i.e., the individual mandate) and permits individuals who receive private health insurance through a plan offered by a tribe to exclude the value of private health insurance benefits received from their calculation of gross income for tax purposes.
>
> Source: CRS analysis of P.L. 94-437 as amended; P.L. 93-638 as amended, I.R.C. §45(A)(c)(6), and P.L. 111-148 as amended.

These three definitions include individuals who are eligible for IHS services, but some individuals may be eligible for IHS services but not meet any of the ACA statutory definitions of an "Indian" or a member of an "Indian Tribe." IHS eligibility is indicated by tribal membership (i.e., meeting the IHS definition of Indian), but certain other individuals are also eligible for IHS services because they

- reside within an IHS health service delivery area, defined as a county where purchased/referred care services are available;
- reside on tax-exempt land or have ownership of property on land for which the federal government has a trust responsibility;
- are recognized as an Indian by the community in which they live;
- actively participate in tribal affairs; or
- meet other relevant factors in keeping with general Bureau of Indian Affairs (BIA) practices in the jurisdiction for determining eligibility.[49]

A non-Indian woman pregnant with an eligible Indian's child would be eligible for care at an IHS-funded facility during the pregnancy and six weeks following birth, as long as paternity is acknowledged.

Most IHS services are intended for members of federally recognized tribes, but UIOs may also provide services to members of terminated tribes— tribes whose federal recognition was withdrawn by statute—or to tribes that states recognize, but are not recognized by the federal government.[50] Members of terminated or state-recognized tribes are not eligible for services at facilities operated by the IHS, an IT, or a TO.

In a July 1, 2013 rule, HHS addressed the concern that some, but not all, IHS-eligible individuals will be exempt from the requirement to maintain health insurance. The rule provided a hardship exemption for individuals who are eligible for IHS services, but are not members of federally recognized tribes, thereby clarifying that these individuals would not be subject to the individual mandate and associated penalties.[51] American Indians and Alaska Natives who are eligible for an exemption because they meet the ACA definition of "Indian" can claim this exemption through the tax filing process or may apply for an exemption through a health insurance exchange. American Indians seeking a hardship exemption must apply through a health insurance exchange.[52]

SSA HEALTH BENEFIT IMPROVEMENTS FOR INDIANS

The ACA amends the SSA to define a number of Indian terms as they are defined in IHCIA Section 4. These terms include IHS, IT, TOs, UIOs, IHPs, and THPs. These definitions apply for Medicare, Medicaid, and CHIP and general provisions included in SSA Title XI.

The ACA includes amendments to the SSA, although these amendments are not included in the "Indian Health Care Improvement" part of the law. Rather, amendments to the SSA are included in Title II, Subtitle K, "Protections for American Indians and Alaska Natives." This subtitle does the following: (1) it designates facilities operated by IHS, an IT, a TO, or a UIO as the payor of last resort notwithstanding federal or state law to the contrary;[53] (2) it includes IHS, ITs, and TOs as entities that are permitted to determine Medicaid and CHIP eligibility; (3) it prohibits cost sharing for Indians whose incomes are at or below 300% of the federal poverty level and who are enrolled in a qualified health benefit plan in the individual market through the exchange (as established by the ACA),[54] and (4) it extends the period for which IHS, IT, and TO services are reimbursed by Medicare Part B for all services, indefinitely, beginning January 1, 2010. Prior to the ACA, authority for these facilities to receive Medicare Part B reimbursements for certain specified services had expired on January 1, 2010. In addition, the ACA, in Title III, amended the Medicare Part D program to permit costs paid by IHS for prescription drugs for Medicare Part D beneficiaries to count toward the beneficiaries' out-of-pocket threshold for catastrophic protection. In order for a Part D beneficiary to receive catastrophic protection, a certain level of out-of-pocket costs must be incurred; prior to the ACA, expenses incurred by IHS, on behalf of a Part D beneficiary, did not count toward this threshold.[55]

End Notes

[1] P.L. 111-148, 124 Stat. 119, as amended.

[2] P.L. 94-437, 90 Stat, 1401, as amended.

[3] On June 28, 2011, the Supreme Court ruled, in National Federation of Independent Business v. Sebelius (NFIB), on the constitutionality of both the ACA-implemented individual mandate, which requires most U.S. residents (beginning in 2014) to carry health insurance or pay a penalty, and the ACA Medicaid expansion. The Court upheld the individual mandate as a constitutional exercise of Congress's authority to levy taxes. The penalty is to be paid by taxpayers when they file their tax returns and enforced by the Internal Revenue Service. In a separate opinion, the Court found that compelling states to participate in the ACA Medicaid expansion—which the Court determined to be essentially a new program—or risk losing their existing federal Medicaid matching funds was coercive and unconstitutional under the Spending Clause of the Constitution and the Tenth Amendment. The Court's remedy for this constitutional violation was to prohibit HHS from penalizing states that choose not to participate in the expansion by withholding any federal matching funds for their existing Medicaid program. However, if a state accepts the new ACA expansion funds (initially a 100% federal match), it must abide by all the expansion coverage rules. Under NFIB, all other provisions of ACA—including the Indian Health Care Improvement Act—remain fully intact and operative.

[4] Other provisions in the ACA may also affect Indian health. For example, Indian tribes may be eligible for new grant or contract programs that augment the health care workforce or improve public health, they may participate in reforms made to the private insurance market, and they may benefit from Medicare and Medicaid reforms. More information about ACA changes can be found at CRS's website under "Issue in Focus-Affordable Care Act and Health Policy" at http://www.crs.gov/Pages/subissue.aspx? cliid=3746&parentid =13.

[5] For more information about the Indian Health Service (IHS), see CRS Report R43330, The Indian Health Service (IHS): An Overview, by Elayne J. Heisler.

[6] IHS provides services to American Indians and Alaska Natives residing in 35 states. Area offices may serve tribes in one state, such as the Alaska Area office that administers services in Alaska, or may serve tribes in multiple states, such as the Nashville Area office that administers services for tribes on the east coast, in Alabama, Louisiana, and parts of Texas.

[7] Self-determination contracts and self-governance compacts are authorized by P.L. 93-638, the Indian Self-Determination and Education Assistance Act of January 4, 1975, 88 Stat. 2203, as amended; 25 U.S.C. §450 et seq.

[8] See 42 C.F.R. §136.11, "Services available;" and CRS Report R43330, The Indian Health Service (IHS): An Overview, by Elayne J. Heisler.

[9] CRS Report R43330, The Indian Health Service (IHS): An Overview, by Elayne J. Heisler.

[10] U.S. Department of Health and Human Services, Indian Health Service, "IHS Fact Sheets: Safe Water and Waste Disposal Facilities," January 2013, http://www.ihs.gov/newsroom/factsheets/safewater/.

[11] In addition to IHCIA, the Snyder Act of 1921 (P.L. 67-85, act of November 2, 1921, 42 Stat. 208, as amended; 25 U.S.C. §13) also authorizes Indian health programs.

[12] P.L. 102-573, act of October 29, 1992, 106 Stat. 4526.

[13] Omnibus Indian Advancement Act, P.L. 106-568, §815, act of December 27, 2000, 114 Stat. 2868, 2918.

Indian Health Care: Impact of the Affordable Care Act (ACA) 89

[14] IHCIA reauthorization bills were introduced in the 106th (H.R. 3397 and S. 2526), 107th (S. 212 and H.R. 1662), 108th (S. 556 and H.R. 2440), 109th (H.R. 5312, S. 1057, S. 3524, and S. 4122), 110th (H.R. 1328, S. 1200, and S. 2532); and 111th (H.R. 2708 and S. 1790) Congresses.

[15] For a discussion of the relationship between appropriations and authorizations, see CRS Report RS20371, Overview of the Authorization-Appropriations Process, by Bill Heniff Jr.

[16] This is S. 1790 in the 111th Congress.

[17] More information about the private health insurance provisions in the ACA can be found in CRS Report R42069, Private Health Insurance Market Reforms in the Patient Protection and Affordable Care Act (ACA), by Annie L. Mach and Bernadette Fernandez, and CRS Report R42663, Health Insurance Exchanges Under the Patient Protection and Affordable Care Act (ACA), by Bernadette Fernandez and Annie L. Mach. In addition, the ACA contains other changes that may affect American Indians and Alaska Natives, but these are not discussed in this report. For Medicare-related changes, see CRS Report R41196, Medicare Provisions in the Patient Protection and Affordable Care Act (PPACA): Summary and Timeline, coordinated by Patricia A. Davis. For information on Medicaid and Children's Health Insurance Program-related provisions, see CRS Report R41210, Medicaid and the State Children's Health Insurance Program (CHIP) Provisions in ACA: Summary and Timeline, by Evelyne P. Baumrucker et al. For public health, workforce, and quality-related changes, see CRS Report R41278, Public Health, Workforce, Quality, and Related Provisions in ACA: Summary and Timeline, coordinated by C. Stephen Redhead and Elayne J. Heisler.

[18] The ACA defines the term "Indian" in three different ways. The three definitions are discussed below in "ACA Private Health Insurance Changes."

[19] 25 U.S.C. §47.

[20] P.L. 93-638 and 25 U.S.C. §§450 et seq.

[21] More information about the Substance Abuse and Mental Health Services Administration (SAMHSA) can be found in CRS Report R43304, Public Health Service Agencies: Overview and Funding, coordinated by Amalia K. Corby-Edwards and C. Stephen Redhead.

[22] Prior to the ACA, IHS was the payor of last resort only for contract health services (CHS) (See 42 C.F.R. §136.61). In general, Medicaid is considered the payor of last resort.

[23] Beginning with the FY2014 budget justification, CHS is now referred to as the purchased/referred care program. See U.S. Dept. of Health and Human Services, Indian Health Service, Fiscal Year 2014 Indian Health Service Justification of Estimates, http://www.ihs.gov/BudgetFormulation/documents/FY2014BudgetJustification.pdf.

[24] U.S. Department of Health and Human Services, Indian Health Service, "IHS Fact Sheets: Workforce," January 2010, http://www.ihs.gov/PublicAffairs/IHSBrochure/Workforce.asp. For more recent information about HIS workforce vacancies, see CRS Report R43330, The Indian Health Service (IHS): An Overview, by Elayne J. Heisler.

[25] These states are Arizona, California, North Dakota, and South Dakota.

[26] Act of March 3, 1931, chap. 411, 71st Cong., 46 Stat. 1494, as amended; 40 U.S.C., Chap. 31, Subchap. IV. The Davis-Bacon Act requires that employers pay prevailing wage rates, as determined by the Secretary of Labor, on federal construction projects. For more information, see CRS Report R41469, Davis-Bacon Prevailing Wages and State Revolving Loan Programs Under the Clean Water Act and the Safe Drinking Water Act, by Gerald Mayer and Jon O. Shimabukuro.

[27] CMS programs are also referred to herein as SSA health benefits programs.

[28] See CRS Report R40444, State Children's Health Insurance Program (CHIP): A Brief Overview, by Elicia J. Herz and Evelyne P. Baumrucker.

[29] In general, Medicaid is a shared federal and state program in which the state government pays a share of Medicaid expenses based on a formula where the federal share is inversely proportional to the state's per capita income (i.e., states with lower per capita income receive a greater percentage of Medicaid payments from the federal government).

[30] A memorandum of understanding between IHS and the VA was signed on October 1, 2010; see http://www.ihs.gov/ announcements/documents/3-OD-11-0006.pdf. See also, U.S. Department of Veterans Affairs, "VA and Indian Health Service Announce National Reimbursement Agreement," press release, December 6, 2012.

[31] The Navajo reservation is located in parts of Arizona, Utah, and New Mexico.

[32] The Snyder Act of 1921 (P.L. 67-85, act of November 2, 1921, 42 Stat. 208, as amended; 25 U.S.C. §13) provides general authorization for Indian health programs. The Snyder Act is a permanent, indefinite authorization for federal Indian programs, including for "conservation of health."

[33] "Terminated" tribes are tribes whose federal recognition was withdrawn by statute.

[34] U.S. Department of Health and Human Services, Indian Health Service, Indian Health Service: Fiscal Year 2012 Justification of Estimates for Appropriations Committees (Rockville, MD: HHS, 2012), http://www.ihs.gov/ NonMedicalPrograms/Budget Formulation/ documents /FY%202012%20Budget%20Justification.pdf

[35] IHS is forbidden to bill or charge Indians (see 25 U.S.C. §1681 and 25 U.S.C. §458aaa-14), but IHCIA, Title V does not prohibit UIHPs from charging their patients.

[36] IHS, Office of Urban Indian Health Programs, Urban Indian Health Program Statistics, FY2005 (Rockville, MD: October 16, 2007), p. 4.

[37] Section 201(a), P.L. 81-152, act of June 30, 1949, 63 Stat. 377, 383, as amended; 40 U.S.C. §501.

[38] For more information on the Public Health Service, see CRS Report R43304, Public Health Service Agencies: Overview and Funding, coordinated by Amalia K. Corby-Edwards and C. Stephen Redhead.

[39] U. S. Government Accountability Office, Indian Health Service: Most American Indians and Alaska Natives Potentially Eligible for Expanded Health Coverage, but Action Needed to Increase Enrollment, 13-533, September 5, 2013, http://www.gao.gov/products/GAO-13-553.

[40] GAO has released four reports on aspects of the CHS program: (1) GAO-11-767, "Indian Health Service: Increased Oversight Needed to Ensure Accuracy of Data Used for Estimating Contract Health Service Need." http://www.gao.gov/new.items/d11767.pdf, September 23, 2011; (2) GAO-12-446, "Indian Health Service: Action Needed to Ensure Equitable Allocation of Resources for the Contract Health Service Program," http://www.gao.gov/ assets/600/591631.pdf, June 15, 2012; (3) GAO 13-272, Indian Health Service: Capping Payments for Nonhospital Services Could Save Millions of Dollars for Contract Health Services, http://www.gao.gov/products/GAO-13-272, April 11, 2013; and (4) GAO 14-57, "Indian Health Service: Opportunities May Exist to Improve the Contract Health Service Program," http://www.gao.gov/products/GAO-14-57, December 11, 2013.

[41] P.L. 100-579, act of October 31, 1988, 102 Stat. 2916, as amended; 42 U.S.C. Chap 122 (§11701 et seq.).

[42] This program receives appropriations through the federal health center program. For more information, see http://bphc.hrsa.gov/about/specialpopulations.htm or CRS Report R42433, Federal Health Centers, by Elayne J. Heisler.

Indian Health Care: Impact of the Affordable Care Act (ACA)   91

[43] For details, see The Indian Health Care Improvement Act Reauthorization and Extension Act of 2009 as Enacted by PPACA: Detailed Summary and Timeline by Elayne J. Heisler. CRS Report R43233, Private Health Plans Under the ACA: In Brief, by Bernadette Fernandez and Annie L. Mach

[44] CRS Report R43233, Private Health Plans Under the ACA: In Brief, by Bernadette Fernandez and Annie L. Mach.

[45] Section 14029(d) in P.L. 111-148; 45 C.F.R. §155.420(d)(8) see CRS Report R41152, Indian Health Care: Impact of the Affordable Care Act (ACA), by Elayne J. Heisler.

[46] Individuals may change plans outside of the general enrollment period if they experience certain qualifying life events (e.g., the birth or adoption of a child or a change in marital status). For more information, 45 C.F.R. §155.420.

[47] CRS Report R41331, Individual Mandate and Related Information Requirements Under ACA, by Annie L. Mach.

[48] Section 9021 excludes the following health benefits from calculations of gross income: (1) health services or benefits provided or purchased by IHS, an IT, or a TO or through programs of third parties funded by the IHS; (2) medical care services, including those provided, purchased, or reimbursed by an IT or TO or to a member of an IT and the member's spouse or dependents; (3) accident or health plan coverage (or an arrangement having the same effect) provided by an IT or TO for medical care to a member of an IT and the member's spouse or dependents; and (4) any other medical care provided by an IT that supplements, replaces, or substitutes for the programs and services provided by the federal government to IT or tribal members.

[49] 42 C.F.R. §136.12(a). The Bureau of Indian Affairs (BIA) is an agency within the U.S. Department of the Interior.

[50] 25 U.S.C. §§1 603(f), 1651-1660d.

[51] Center for Medicare & Medicaid Services, "Patient Protection and Affordable Care Act; Exchange Functions: Eligibility for Exemptions; Miscellaneous Minimum Essential Coverage Provisions; Final Rule," 78 Federal Register 39494-39529, July 1, 2013.

[52] U.S. Department of Health and Human Services, Indian Health Service, "The Affordable Care Act and the Indian Health Service," http://www.ihs.gov/ACA/. Individuals eligible for a hardship exemption may also be eligible for catastrophic health insurance plans. For more information, see CRS Report R42663, Health Insurance Exchanges Under the Patient Protection and Affordable Care Act (ACA), by Bernadette Fernandez and Annie L. Mach.

[53] Prior to the ACA, IHS was the payor of last resort only for contract health services (CHS) (See 42 C.F.R. §136.61). In general, Medicaid is considered the payor of last resort.

[54] This applies to private insurance coverage and is also discussed above; see "ACA Private Health Insurance Changes."

[55] See Section 3114 in CRS Report R41196, Medicare Provisions in the Patient Protection and Affordable Care Act (PPACA): Summary and Timeline, coordinated by Patricia A. Davis.

In: The Indian Health Service
Editor: Pamela M. Agnelli

ISBN: 978-1-63321-582-5
© 2014 Nova Science Publishers, Inc.

Chapter 4

THE INDIAN HEALTH CARE IMPROVEMENT ACT REAUTHORIZATION AND EXTENSION AS ENACTED BY THE ACA: DETAILED SUMMARY AND TIMELINE[*]

Elayne J. Heisler

SUMMARY

On March 23, 2010, President Obama signed into law a comprehensive health care reform bill, the Patient Protection and Affordable Care Act (ACA; P.L. 111-148). Among its provisions, the ACA reenacts, amends, and permanently reauthorizes the Indian Health Care Improvement Act (IHCIA). IHCIA authorizes many specific Indian Health Service (IHS) activities, sets out the national policy for health services administered to Indians, and sets health condition goals for the IHS service population to reduce "the prevalence and incidence of preventable illnesses among, and unnecessary and premature deaths of, Indians." The reauthorization of IHCIA in the ACA amends the IHCIA to, among other changes, expand programs that seek to augment the IHS health care workforce, increase the amount and type of services available at facilities funded by the IHS, and increase the number and type of

---

[*] This is an edited, reformatted and augmented version of a Congressional Research Service publication, No. R41630, dated January 3, 2014.

programs that provide behavioral health and substance abuse treatment to American Indians and Alaska Natives.

This report provides a brief overview of IHCIA and summarizes the provisions of the Indian Health Care Improvement Reauthorization and Extension Act of 2009 as enacted and amended by Section 10221 of the ACA. **Appendix A** presents a timeline of the deadlines included in the act.

This report is primarily for reference purposes. The material in it is intended to provide context to help the reader better understand the intent of ACA's individual provisions at the time of enactment. The report does not track or discuss ongoing ACA-related regulatory and other implementation activities.

INTRODUCTION

On March 23, 2010, President Obama signed into law a comprehensive health care reform bill, the Patient Protection and Affordable Care Act (ACA; P.L. 111-148).[1] Among its provisions, the ACA creates a mandate for most U.S. residents to obtain health insurance and provides for the establishment of insurance exchanges through which certain individuals and families will be able to receive federal subsidies to reduce the cost of purchasing that coverage. The new law expands eligibility for Medicaid; amends the Medicare program in ways that are intended to reduce the growth in Medicare spending that had been projected under preexisting law; imposes an excise tax on insurance plans determined to have high premiums; and makes other changes to the federal tax code, Medicare, Medicaid, and numerous other programs.[2] The ACA also reenacts, amends, and permanently reauthorizes the Indian Health Care Improvement Act (IHCIA).[3] Specifically, Section 10221(a) of the ACA enacted the Indian Health Care Improvement Reauthorization and Extension Act of 2009 (S. 1790)[4] (hereinafter referred to as the IHCIA Reauthorization and Extension Act). Section 10221(b) of the ACA amended sections of the IHCIA Reauthorization and Extension Act (e.g., Sections 111, 134, and 201) and amended one section of IHCIA not included in the IHCIA Reauthorization and Extension Act (Section 806). Another report, *Indian Health Care: Impact of the Affordable Care Act (ACA)*, by Elayne J. Heisler, more briefly summarizes the major changes made by the ACA to IHCIA and includes a discussion of other provisions in the ACA that may affect the Indian Health Service (IHS), American Indian and Alaska Native health, and their access to health care.

IHCIA authorizes many specific IHS activities, sets out the national policy for health services administered to Indians, and sets health condition goals for the IHS service population to reduce "the prevalence and incidence of preventable illnesses among, and unnecessary and premature deaths of, Indians."[5] Prior to the ACA, IHCIA was last fully reauthorized by the Indian Health Amendments of 1992,[6] which extended authorizations of its appropriations through FY2000. The authorizations for all IHCIA programs were later extended through FY2001.[7] Although authority had expired, IHCIA authorized programs continued to receive annual appropriations since FY2001.

OVERVIEW OF INDIAN HEALTH CARE[8]

The IHS, an agency within the Department of Health and Human Services (HHS), provides health care for approximately 2.2 million eligible American Indians/Alaska Natives through a system of programs and facilities located on or near Indian reservations, and through contractors in certain urban areas.[9] IHS provides services in 35 states, subdivided into 12 geographic "Areas" that consist of one or more states.[10] Each Area is administered by an Area Office; Areas, in turn, are further subdivided into service units that consist of one or more facilities. IHS may provide services directly, or Indian tribes (ITs) or tribal organizations (TOs) may operate IHS facilities and programs themselves through self-determination contracts and self-governance compacts negotiated with IHS.[11] Although most IHS facilities are located on or near reservations, IHS also funds urban Indian health projects (UIHPs), through grants or contracts to urban Indian organizations (UIOs).

The IHCIA authorizes many specific IHS activities, sets out the national policy for health services administered to Indians, and declares that one of the federal goals for the health condition of the IHS service population is to "provide the quantity and quality of health services that will permit the health status of Indians to be raised to the highest possible level."[12] Significantly, IHCIA authorizes direct collections from Medicare, Medicaid, and other third-party insurers. IHCIA also gave IHS authority to grant funding to UIOs, authorized programs to expand the health care workforce providing services at IHS-funded facilities, and authorized programs that address health concerns for the American Indian and Alaska Native population (e.g., substance abuse, suicide, diabetes).

OVERVIEW OF REPORT

This report summarizes the provisions of the IHCIA Reauthorization and Extension Act as enacted by Section 10221 of the ACA.[13] This report is primarily for reference purposes. The material in it is intended to provide context to help the reader understand the intent of the ACA's individual provisions at the time of enactment. The act includes two titles. Title I contains amendments to the eight IHCIA titles. Title II amends and reauthorizes the Native Hawaiian Health Care Act,[14] which authorizes health education, health promotion, disease prevention services, and health professions scholarship programs for Native Hawaiians.[15] This report focuses on Title I, which contains eight sections, each of which amends a specific IHCIA Title. Title I also, with some exceptions, consolidates IHCIA appropriations into a single section, repealing authorizations that had previously been included at the end of each of IHCIA's eight titles. The section numbers below refer to the section numbers in the IHCIA Reauthorization and Extension Act. Where appropriate, sections amended by Section 10221(b) of the ACA are noted. The subtitles below refer to those in the IHCIA Reauthorization and Extension Act, which correspond to the IHCIA title they amend. Each subtitle begins with some background on the IHCIA title it amends to provide context for the descriptions of the law's provisions. This background reflects the policy issues at the time of enactment and does not reflect the effects of the ACA. **Table 1** describes the major differences between the IHCIA and the IHCIA Reauthorization Extension Act.

Appendix A includes a detailed timeline of effective dates for the IHCIA Reauthorization and Extension Act provisions. Appendix B includes a list of acronyms used in this report. The term "Secretary," as used in this report, means the Secretary of HHS, unless otherwise indicated. The term "Indian" in this report refers to "Indian" as defined in IHCIA. Under this definition, an Indian is a person who is a member of a federally recognized tribe, band, nation, or other organized group or community, including any Alaska Native village or group, or regional or village corporation, as defined in or established pursuant to the Alaska Native Claims Settlement Act.[16] The ACA also defined a number of new Indian-related terms. Two of the new terms most frequently used in this report are Indian Health Program and Tribal Health Program. "Indian Health Program" (IHP) is defined as (1) any health program administered by the IHS, (2) any Tribal Health Program, or (3) any Indian tribe or tribal organization to which the Secretary provides funding under the Buy Indian Act. "Tribal Health Program" (THP) is defined as any IT or TO

The Indian Health Care Improvement Act Reauthorization ... 97

operating any health program, service, function, activity, or facility funded, in whole or part, by the IHS through, or provided for in, a contract or compact with the IHS under the Indian Self-Determination and Education Assistance Act (ISDEAA).[17]

Table 1. IHCIA Reauthorization Summary

IHCIA Title Name and Subject	ACA
Title I-Indian Health Manpower Authorizes workforce programs to increase the supply of providers at IHS facilities	Maintains title's major sections; repeals section authorizing appropriations for the title; expands use of community health aide workers at IHS-funded facilities; adds a new section funding a demonstration to address IHS health professional shortages; and exempts employees at IHS-funded facilities from certain licensing, registration requirements and related fees.
Title II-Health Services Authorizes IHS health services, research, payments for service-related transportation, payment for services provided through contracts with outside providers (i.e., Contract Health Services (CHS))	Maintains title's major sections; repeals section authorizing appropriations for the title; amends authorization for two funds (Indian Health Care Improvement Fund and Catastrophic Health Emergency Fund); expands IHS authority for diabetes, cancer screening, and long-term care programs; and amends sections related to the CHS program.
Title III-Health Facilities Authorizes construction and renovation of IHS facilities; sets procedures by which construction and renovation projects are selected	Maintains title's major sections; repeals section authorizing appropriations for the title; amends IHS construction priority system; and adds new sections requiring grants to build modular and mobile facilities.
Title IV-Access to Health Services	Maintains title's major sections; repeals section authorizing appropriations for the title; adds the State Children's Health Insurance Program to programs that IHS is authorized to bill;

Table 1. (Continued)

IHCIA Title Name and Subject	ACA
Authorizes IHS programs to bill Medicare, Medicaid, and private insurance	adds new sections permitting ITs, TOs, and UIOS to purchase federal employee health and life insurance benefits for their employees; expands IHS collaboration with the Department of Veterans Affairs and the Department of Defense.
Title V-Health Services for Urban Indians Authorizes grants to UIOs for health projects to serve urban Indians	Maintains title's major sections; repeals section authorizing appropriations for the title; expands grant opportunities available to UIOs.
Title VI-Organization Improvements Establishes IHS's organizational position within HHS; the position of Director of IHS; and requires an automated management information system for IHS record-keeping	Maintains title's major sections; establishes that the IHS Director should report directly to the HHS Secretary; adds new sections requiring: (1) an Office of Direct Service Tribes; and (2) a plan to create a new Nevada Area Office.
Title VII-Behavioral Health Programs Authorizes programs related to behavioral health prevention and treatment	Replaces IHCIA Title VII with new language authorizing new comprehensive behavioral health and treatment programs. Includes a new subsection authorizing programs related to youth suicide prevention.
Title VIII-Miscellaneous Requires the IHS Director to submit a number of reports; establishes IHS eligibility for health services; and defines California Indians, amongst other provisions	Maintains title's major sections; repeals section authorizing appropriations for the title; adds new sections that, among other things, establish (1) a prescription drugs monitoring program; (2) an IHS Director of HIV/AIDS Prevention and Treatment; and (3) new requirements for the IHS budget requests to reflect inflation and changes in the IHS service population.

Source: CRS analysis of P.L. 94-437, as amended (IHCIA), and P.L. 111-148 (ACA).

The Indian Health Care Improvement Act Reauthorization ...   99

TITLE I—IHCIA REAUTHORIZATION AND AMENDMENTS

Subtitle A—Indian Health Manpower[18]

Subtitle A includes sections that amend IHCIA Title I "Indian Health Manpower." This title includes provisions related to personnel recruitment, scholarships, and other educational programs that seek to augment the Indian health workforce. IHS had high vacancy rates in many of its health professions—25% for physicians, 15% for dentists, and 16% for nurses, for instance, as of January 2010.[19] These vacancy rates are higher than those of federally funded health centers in rural areas, facilities that also have a difficult time recruiting providers.[20] The purpose of IHCIA Title I is to increase the number, and also enhance the skills, of Indian and non-Indian health professionals and other health personnel in the IHS.

The ACA maintains a number of existing sections that authorize scholarships for preparatory and professional schools. It also authorizes new programs that may expand the workforce at IHS, IT, TO, and UIO facilities. Specifically, it authorizes programs that may expand the use of community health workers outside of Alaska, may increase the number of providers at facilities with severe shortages, and it amends licensing requirements for UIO providers to facilitate UIOs provider recruitment.

Section 111. Community Health Aide Program[21]

This section amends **IHCIA Section 119** [25 U.S.C. §1616l] with new language that requires the Secretary, under authority of the Snyder Act,[22] to develop and operate a Community Health Aide Program (CHAP) in Alaska, under which IHS is to train Alaska Natives to provide health care, health promotion, and disease prevention in rural Alaska Native villages. The section requires the Secretary to provide, in a specified manner, a high standard of training to community health aides; establish teleconferencing capacity in health clinics located in or near those villages for use of CHAPs or community health practitioners; establish and maintain a CHAP certification board; and provide continuing education, close supervision, and a system to review and evaluate CHAP work. The section also prohibits a CHAP dental health aide therapist from performing certain pulpal therapy or extractions without a determination of a medical emergency by a licensed dentist and from performing any other oral or jaw surgeries except for uncomplicated extractions.

The section requires the Secretary, acting through IHS, to establish a neutral review panel to study the CHAP dental health aide therapist program to ensure that the quality of care is adequate and appropriate. The section specifies panel membership, the factors of the study, and requires consultation with Alaska tribal organizations, and a report to Congress.

The section also authorizes the expansion of CHAP, except for the dental health aide therapist program, into a national program, but requires that the expansion not reduce Alaska CHAP funding. The section exempts ITs and TOs using dental health aides from certain specified instructional requirements for ITs or TOs located in states (other than Alaska) that permit, under state law, dental health aide therapists or midlevel health providers to supply such services. The section requires the Secretary, acting through the IHS, to facilitate the implementation of dental health aide programs by ITs and TOs who elect to provide these services; and prohibits the Secretary from filling IHS program vacancies for certified dentists with dental health aides. The section further specifies that nothing in this section restricts the ability of IHS, an IT, or a TO to participate in any program or to provide any service authorized in any other federal law.

Section 112. Health Professional Chronic Shortage Demonstration Programs

This section adds a new **IHCIA Section 123** *Health Professional Chronic Shortage Demonstration Programs* [25 U.S.C. §1616p], which authorizes the Secretary, acting through IHS, to fund demonstration programs for IHPs to address chronic shortages of health professionals. The section specifies the purposes of the demonstration programs, and requires that the program incorporate an advisory board composed of representatives from tribes, IHPs, and Indian communities served by the program.

Section 113. Exemption from Payment of Certain Fees

This section adds a new **IHCIA Section 124** *Exemption of Payment of Certain Fees* [25 U.S.C. §1616q], which exempts employees of a THP or UIO from the payment of licensing, registration, and other fees imposed by a federal agency, to the same extent that Public Health Service (PHS) Commissioned Corps officers or other IHS employees are exempt from the fees.

Subtitle B—Health Services

Subtitle B includes sections that amend IHCIA Title II "Health Services" authorizing a number of specific non-behavioral health programs and activities, including prevention activities, diabetes and cancer programs, Indian men's health, Indian school health education programs, research and epidemiological centers, and a fund for the elimination of funding inequities among health care programs. The ACA amends a number of programs in this title. It also authorizes a report that studies and makes recommendations about contract health service (CHS)[23] funding and how IHS funding is distributed across IHS service areas. CHS refers to services that IHS, ITs, or TOs may purchase, through contract, from private providers in instances where the THP cannot provide the needed care.

Section 121. Indian Health Care Improvement Fund

This section amends **IHCIA Section 201** [25 U.S.C. §1621] with new language that authorizes the Secretary, acting through IHS, to use funds designated as the "Indian Health Care Improvement Fund" (IHCIF), to eliminate tribes' deficiencies in health status and resources (as defined in the section), eliminate backlogs in provision of health care to Indians, meet health needs efficiently and equitably, eliminate inequities in funding for both direct care and CHS, and augment the ability of IHS to meet 10 specified health service responsibilities. The Secretary is authorized to expend IHCIF funds either directly or through contracts or compacts under ISDEAA. The section also prohibits using funds appropriated under this section to offset funds appropriated under other laws, permits IHCIF allocation among service units and THPs, and requires the Secretary to determine (in consultation with the affected ITs and TOs) the apportionment of funds among service units, ITs, and TOs for the specified health service responsibilities. The section also requires that THPs be equally eligible for funds with IHS programs and requires that appropriations under this section be included in the base budget of the IHS for subsequent fiscal years. The section requires the Secretary to submit a report to Congress three years after enactment on the current health status and resource deficiencies for each tribe or service unit, and specifies the data to be included in this report. In addition, the section specifies that nothing in the section is intended to diminish the primary responsibility of the IHS to eliminate backlogs in unmet health care or to discourage additional efforts by IHS to achieve parity among tribes.

Section 122. Catastrophic Health Emergency Fund

This section replaces **IHCIA Section 202** [25 U.S.C. §1621a] with new language that establishes the Catastrophic Health Emergency Fund (CHEF), administered by the Secretary through IHS headquarters, to meet extraordinary medical costs associated with the treatment of victims of disasters or catastrophic illnesses. The section specifies the uses, administration, and regulations of this fund. It also specifies that CHEF consists of appropriations and third-party reimbursements to which IHS is entitled for treatments paid for by CHEF, and requires that no part of the CHEF or the administration thereof be subject to contract or grant (including those made under ISDEAA). It prohibits CHEF from being apportioned on an Area Office, Service Unit, or any other basis. The section also prohibits funds appropriated to CHEF from being used to offset or limit other IHS appropriations and it requires that all reimbursements to which IHS is entitled from any source, by reason of treatment rendered to any victim of a disaster or catastrophic illness, the cost of which was paid from CHEF, be deposited into CHEF.

Section 123. Diabetes Prevention, Treatment, and Control

This section inserts a new **IHCIA Section 204** *Diabetes Prevention, Treatment, and Control* [25 U.S.C. §1621c], which requires the Secretary, acting through IHS and in consultation with ITs and TOs, to determine the incidence of diabetes and its complications among Indians and, based on the incidence determined, what actions IHS service units need to take to prevent, treat, and control the disease, including effective ongoing monitoring. The Secretary is required—to the extent indicated and with medical consent—to screen Indians for diabetes and for conditions that indicate a high risk for diabetes. The section also permits screening through Internet-based programs, and requires the Secretary to establish a cost-effective approach to ensure ongoing monitoring of diabetes indicators. In addition, the Secretary is required to maintain model diabetes projects in existence at enactment, and is required to provide recurring funding to ITs and THPs for diabetes projects that these entities operate under this section, including funding for projects in existence at enactment and funded thereafter.

In addition, the section authorizes the Secretary to provide dialysis programs for IHS, ITs, and TOs, including equipment and staffing. The Secretary is also required to consult with the ITs and TOs in each IHS area on diabetes programs, establish diabetes patient registries in each IHS Area Office, and ensure that the data collected are disseminated to other Area Offices. The section also authorizes diabetes control officers in each IHS Area

The Indian Health Care Improvement Act Reauthorization ...

Office and states that any activity carried out by a diabetes control officer that is the subject of a contract or compact of ISDEAA, and any funds made available to carry out these activities may not be divisible for the purposes of ISDEAA.

Section 124. Other Authority for Provision of Services and Long-Term Care

This section inserts a new **IHCIA Section 205** [25 U.S.C. §1621d], which authorizes the Secretary to provide funding, through programs and services of IHS, ITs, and TOs, for healthcare-related services and programs (not otherwise specified in IHCIA) for hospice care, assisted living, long-term care, and home- and community-based services (as defined in this section). The section also specifies eligibility criteria for long-term care services, authorizes funding through IHS, ITs, and TOs, for "convenient care services" pursuant to IHCIA Section 307(c)(2)(A), and repeals IHCIA Section 821, which had authorized a demonstration for home-and community based services.

This section also amends **IHCIA Section 822** [25 U.S.C. §1680l] by authorizing the Secretary, acting through the IHS, to provide, directly or through ISDEAA contracts or compacts with THPs, long-term care and health care services associated with long-term care at any long-term care or related facility owned or operated by a THP directly or under ISDEAA. The section requires that the agreements provide for sharing staff and other services between an IHS facility and the contracting IT's or TO's facility. The section authorizes such contracts to allow delegation to the contractors of necessary supervision over IHS employees, and permits ITs and TOs to construct, renovate, or expand nursing facilities. The section also specifies certain terms of the agreement, including funding allocations, and specifies that any nursing facility funded under this section must meet the requirements for such facilities under Medicare statute. The section requires the Secretary to provide necessary technical and other assistance to tribal applicants, and encourages the use of existing underused facilities and permits the use of swing beds, for longterm or similar care.

Section 125 Third Parties Reimbursements

This section amends **IHCIA Section 206** [25 U.S.C. §1621e] by inserting new language that permits the United States, ITs, and TOs the right to recover reasonable charges billed (or, if higher, the highest amount a third party would pay for care and services from a non-governmental provider) for health services provided by these entities to an individual, to the same extent that the individual or any nongovernmental provider of health services would be eligible to receive reimbursement or indemnification. The section specifies that entities from whom recovery can occur include insurance companies, health maintenance organizations, employee benefit plans, third-party tortfeasors, state political subdivisions, local governments, or any other responsible or liable third parties. The section limits the right of recovery against any state to circumstances where the health services are covered under workers' compensation laws or a no-fault automobile accident insurance plan. The section prohibits state or local laws, contract provisions, insurance or health maintenance organization policies, employee benefit plans, self-insurance plans, managed care plans, or other health care plans or programs entered into or renewed after November 23, 1988, from preventing or hindering the right of recovery. The section also prohibits any action by the United States, an IT, or a TO from affecting the right of an injured person to collect for the portion of their damages not covered hereunder. In addition, the section permits the United States, an IT, or a TO to enforce the right of recovery by intervening or joining in specified civil actions or proceedings, or by instituting a separate civil action (after notifying the individual or his representatives or heirs), and requires reasonable efforts to notify the individual.

The section also authorizes ITs or TOs, independent of the rights of the injured or diseased person, to recover from tortfeasors or their insurers the reasonable value of health services provided or paid in accordance with the Federal Medical Care Recovery Act.

The section prohibits the United States from recovering from an IT's, TO's, or UIO's self-insurance plan, but allows recovery from a tribe if the tribal governing body provides specific written authorization for a specified time period and permits expenditure of amounts recovered to provide additional health services. The section requires the awarding of reasonable attorney fees and costs of litigation to prevailing plaintiffs under this section, prohibits specified health insurance and related entities from denying reimbursement of an IHS or IT's or TO's claim on the basis of the claim's format (if the format meets certain standards), and applies a specified statute of limitations.[24] The section applies to UIOs the same rights of recovery, for the populations they serve, as those allowed to ITs and TOs for their served populations. The section also provides that nothing in it limits the right of the United States, an IT, or a TO to recover under any applicable federal, state, or tribal law, including medical lien laws.

Section 126. Crediting of Reimbursements

This section amends **IHCIA Section 207** [25 U.S.C. §1621f] with language that requires that— except as provided under IHCIA Section 202 regarding the CHEF or under IHCIA Section 813 regarding services to ineligible persons—all reimbursements received or recovered for provision of health service by IHS, an IT, a TO, or a UIO are required to be credited to the respective entity (including the service unit providing the health service). The section requires that reimbursements be used as specified under IHCIA Section 401 ("Section 151. Treatment of Payments under SSA Health Benefits Programs"). The section also prohibits IHS from offsetting or limiting the amounts obligated to any service unit, or any entity receiving IHS funding, because of the receipt of reimbursements under this section.

Section 127. Behavioral Health Training and Community Education Programs

This section amends **IHCIA Section 209** [25 U.S.C. §1621h] by inserting new language requiring the HHS Secretary, acting through IHS, and the Secretary of the Interior, in consultation with IT and TOs, to conduct a study and compile a list of specified types of staff positions within the Bureau of Indian Affairs (BIA), IHS, ITs, and TOs, whose qualifications should include training in the identification, prevention, education, referral, or treatment of mental illness, dysfunction, or self-destructive behavior. The appropriate secretary is required to provide culturally relevant training criteria appropriate for each type of position and to ensure that this training has been or will be provided. IHS is also required, upon request by a IT, TO, or UIO, to develop and implement a program of community education on mental illness, or assist the requester with doing so. The section specifies that when the positions are funded under ISDEAA the appropriate secretary is required to ensure that training costs are included in the contract or compact. The section also requires the IHS to provide technical assistance for obtaining and developing community education materials. Within 90 days of enactment, the HHS Secretary is required to develop a plan, to be implemented under the Snyder Act, to increase behavioral health services by at least 500 staff positions within five years, with at least 200 of such positions devoted to child, adolescent, and family services.

Section 128. Cancer Screening

This section amends **IHCIA Section 212** [25 U.S.C. §1621k] by adding that mammography be provided under standards established by the Secretary under the SSA, to ensure the safety and accuracy of the mammography and other cancer screenings.

Section 129. Patient Travel Costs

This section amends **IHCIA Section 213** [25 U.S.C. §1621l] to insert new language that authorizes the Secretary, through IHS, to provide funds for specified patient travel costs associated with receiving IHS-funded health care services (those provided directly by IHS or through ISDEAA contract or compact). These services include emergency air transport and non-emergency air transport where ground transport is not feasible; transportation by ambulance, specially equipped vehicle, or private vehicle where no other transportation is available; or other means required when air or motor vehicle transport is not available. The section also authorizes the Secretary to provide funding for qualified escorts, as defined in the section.

Section 130. Epidemiology Centers

This section amends **IHCIA Section 214** [25 U.S.C. §1621m] with new language that requires the Secretary to establish an epidemiology center in each IHS Area to carry out seven specified functions, in consultation with ITs, TOs, or UIOs. The section specifies that an epidemiology center is subject to ISDEAA. The section also requires that the Director of the Centers for Disease Control and Prevention (CDC) provide technical assistance to these epidemiology centers. The section also authorizes the Secretary to make grants to ITs, TOs, and UIOs, and eligible intertribal consortia (as defined) to operate an epidemiology center and to conduct epidemiological studies of Indian communities, and specifies the criteria for applicants and the uses of such grants. The section further requires that epidemiology centers operated under such grants be treated as public health authorities for purposes of the Health Insurance Portability and Accountability Act[25] (HIPAA). In addition, the section requires the Secretary to grant such centers access to and use of data, data sets, monitoring systems, delivery systems, and other protected health information in the Secretary's possession, and specifies that such centers' activities are, for purposes of HIPAA, for research or disease prevention and control.

Section 131. Indian Youth Grant Program

This section amends **IHCIA Section 216(b)(2)** [25 U.S.C. §1621o] by striking reference to Section 209(m) regarding prohibited uses of grant funds

The Indian Health Care Improvement Act Reauthorization ...   107

and inserts reference to Section 708(c), regarding intermediate adolescent behavioral health services ("Section 708. Indian Youth Program").

Section 132. American Indians into Psychology program

This section amends **IHCIA Section 217** [25 U.S.C. §1621p] by replacing it with new language that authorizes the Secretary, acting through the IHS director, to establish a grant program to award grants of not more than $300,000 to nine colleges and universities for developing and maintaining Indian psychology career recruitment programs. The section requires that one grant be awarded to the University of North Dakota to establish a *Quentin N. Burdick American Indians into Psychology Program*. The section also requires that grants be awarded to locations throughout the United States to maximize their availability to Indian students, including awarding grants to locations that had not previously operated programs. In addition, the section requires the Secretary to issue regulations for competitive funding, and specifies conditions of the grants, including recipients' service obligations. The section authorizes to be appropriated $2.7 million for FY2010 and for each fiscal year thereafter.

Section 133. Projects Related to Communicable and Infectious Diseases

This section strikes **IHCIA Section 218** [25 U.S.C. §1621q] replacing it with new language that authorizes the Secretary to make grants to ITs and TOs for projects to prevent, control, and eliminate communicable and infectious diseases, provide public information and education on such diseases, provide education and skills improvement activities on such diseases for health professionals, and establish demonstration projects for the screening, treatment, and prevention of the hepatitis C virus. Grant recipients are encouraged to coordinate their activities with the CDC and state and local health agencies. The section also authorizes the Secretary to provide technical assistance, upon request, and requires the Secretary to make a biennial report to Congress.

Section 134. Licensing[26]

This section amends **IHCIA Section 221** [25 U.S.C. §1621t] to exempt licensed health care professionals from state licensing requirements while employed by a THP providing services under an ISDEAA contract or compact.

This section also amends **IHCIA Section 106** [25 U.S.C. §1615] to insert new language that authorizes the Secretary to provide programs or allowances to encourage specified health professionals and scholarship and stipend recipients under IHCIA Sections 104 (Indian health professions scholarships), 105 (IHS extern programs), 106 (Community Education Allowances), and 115 (Health Training Programs for Community Colleges) to join or continue in an IHP, and to work in rural or remote areas where significant numbers of Indians reside. These programs or allowances include licensing and board or certification examination assistance that may be used to help individuals to transition into IHPs. The section also authorizes the Secretary to provide technical assistance to these health professionals to assist them with fulfilling their service obligations. The section also authorizes programs and allowances for IHS and tribal health professionals to take leave of their duty stations for a period of time each year for specified continuing professional education.

Reauthorization, Findings, and Definitions

Section 101. Reauthorization

This section amends **IHCIA Section 825** [25 U.S.C. §1680o] with new language that authorizes an appropriation of such sums as may be necessary to carry out IHCIA for FY2010 and each fiscal year thereafter to remain available until expended. The section also repeals separate authorizations of appropriations that had been included in each IHCIA title. In addition, it reauthorizes IHCIA indefinitely.

Section 102. Findings

This section amends **IHCIA Section 2** [25 U.S.C. §1601] by adding a new congressional finding that states that providing resources, processes, and structure to eradicate health disparities between Indians and the general population, and that raising Indian health to the highest level are major national goals.

Section 103. Declaration of National Indian Health Policy

This section amends **IHCIA Section 3** [25 U.S.C. §1602] with new language that states that Congress declares that it is the policy of this nation, in fulfillment of special responsibilities and legal obligations to Indians to (1) ensure the highest possible health status for Indians and urban Indians and to provide all resources necessary to effect that policy; (2) raise Indian and urban Indian health status to that set forth in the Healthy People 2010 or successor objectives; (3) ensure maximum Indian participation in the direction of health care services so as to render the persons administering such services and the

The Indian Health Care Improvement Act Reauthorization ... 109

services themselves more responsive to the needs and desires of Indian communities; (4) increase the proportion of all degrees in the health professions and allied and associated professions awarded to Indians so that the proportion of Indian health professionals is the same as the general population in each IHS area; (5) require all actions under this act to be carried out with active and meaningful consultation with ITs and TOs, and conference with UIOs to Indian self-determination; (6) ensure the United States and ITs work in a government-to-government relationship to ensure quality health care for all tribal members; and (7) fund IT and TO-operated programs and facilities at the same level as IHS-operated programs and facilities.

Section 104. Definitions

This section amends **IHCIA Section 4** [25 U.S.C. §1604] by renumbering certain subsections and paragraphs related to specified definitions. The section maintains 12 IHCIA definitions (Area office; fetal alcohol effects; health profession; Indians or Indian; Indian tribe; Secretary; service; service area; substance abuse; urban center; Urban Indian; Urban Indian Organization), amends definitions for 5 terms (disease prevention, fetal alcohol syndrome (FAS), health promotion, service unit, and tribal organization), and adds 12 new terms, for a total of 29 terms. The 12 new terms are "behavioral health," "California Indians," "community college," "contract health service," "Department," "Indian Health Program," "junior or community college," "reservation," "telehealth," "telemedicine," "tribal college or university," and "Tribal Health Program."

This report uses the following terms, as they are used in the IHCIA Reauthorization and Extension Act, to refer to different types of Indian facilities that are eligible for a given program: "Indian Health Program" (IHP), which is defined as any health program administered by the IHS or by an IT or TO under either the Indian Self-Determination and Education Assistance Act, as amended (ISDEAA),[27] or the Buy Indian Act;[28] and "Tribal Health Program" (THP), which is defined as any IT or TO operating a health program under ISDEAA. THPs are included within the term IHP.

Section 135. Liability for Payment

This section amends **IHCIA Section 222** [25 U.S.C. §1621u] to exempt a patient who receives IHS-authorized CHS from being held liable for any charges or costs associated with those authorized services. The section also requires the Secretary to notify, within five business days of the provider receiving a claim, the CHS provider and the patient who receives the services that the patient is not liable for the claim. The section prohibits the CHS provider from recourse against the patient for payment if the notice has been received or if the claim has been deemed accepted under IHCIA Section 220(b) (CHS claims that IHS failed to respond to in the allotted time).

Section 136. Offices of Indian Men's Health and Indian Women's Health

This section amends **IHCIA Section 223** [25 U.S.C. §1621v] to insert new language that authorizes the Secretary, acting through IHS, to establish an office within IHS known as the "Office of Indian Men's Health." The section specifies that a director heads the office and coordinates and promotes the health status of Indian men in the United States. The section requires that the Secretary, acting through IHS, submit a report to Congress describing the activities carried out by the director and any findings with respect to the health of Indian men. The section also requires the Secretary, acting through IHS, to establish an "Office of Indian Women's Health" to monitor and improve the quality of Indian women's health of all ages.

Section 137. CHS Administration and Disbursement Formula

This section adds a new **IHCIA Section 226** *Contract Health Service Administration and Disbursement Formula* [25 U.S.C. §1621y], which requires the Government Accountability Office (GAO) to submit a report, as soon as practicable after enactment, to specified congressional committees and the Secretary, and make it available to each IT, regarding specified elements of the CHS program. Upon receipt of the report, the Secretary is required to consult with ITs regarding the program, including its funding distribution, to determine the adequacy of the current funding formula, and any modifications that are required for the program to be funded at such level as GAO may recommend.[29] The Secretary is authorized, following this consultation, to initiate procedures to negotiate or promulgate regulations to establish a disbursement formula for future CHS program funding.

Subtitle C—Health Facilities

Subtitle C includes sections that amend IHCIA Title III "Health Facilities." This title includes sections related to health care and sanitation facilities. IHS funds the construction, equipping, and maintenance of hospitals, health centers, clinics, and other health care delivery facilities operated by IHS

The Indian Health Care Improvement Act Reauthorization ... 111

and tribes. IHS also funds the construction of water supply and sewage facilities and solid waste disposal systems, and provides technical assistance for the operation and maintenance of such facilities.

The ACA sets new requirements for the priority system for building and renovating facilities and new requirements for closure of IHS-operated health care facilities. It also authorizes demonstration projects to increase the number of facilities available to provide services to American Indians and Alaska Natives including demonstration projects for funding mobile and modular health facilities—two mechanisms considered to build health facilities more rapidly. As discussed below, IHS maintains a priority system to determine which facilities will be built and in what order. The agency also notes that due to funding constraints some facility construction or renovation projects are completed in phases, which may delay completion and increase costs.[30]

Section 141. Health Care Facilities Priority System

This section amends **IHCIA Section 301** [25 U.S.C. §1631] to require the Secretary, acting through IHS, to maintain a health care facility priority system developed in consultation with ITs and TOs that prioritizes tribal needs, includes the methodology for prioritization, and allows for the nomination of new projects at least once every three years. The priority list may also include the top 10 priority facilities for four specified types of facilities as well as other facilities or needs that IHS may identify. The section requires that the Secretary ensure that the planning, design, construction, renovation, and expansion of facilities operated under ISDEAA are fully and equitably integrated into the health care facility priority system. The section also prohibits a project's priority in effect at enactment from being affected by a new facility priority system if the project meets specified criteria and was identified in the FY2008 IHS budget justification as being in the top 10 for four specified types of facilities.[31]

The section also defines the Facilities Appropriations Advisory Board and a Facilities Needs Assessment Workgroup,[32] and requires—not later than one year after enactment—the Secretary to submit to specified committees of Congress an initial report with a national ranked list of all IHS, IT, and TO health care facilities needs developed for the board and workgroup, and requires the Secretary to update the report every five years beginning in 2011. The section also requires the Secretary to submit to the President, for inclusion in reports to Congress,[33] an annual report describing the new health care facility priority system and its methodology, and listing top 10 facilities for four specified types of facilities with justifications and projected costs. The

Secretary is required to prepare this annual report in consultation with ITs, TOs, and UIOs and is required to review the ITs' and TOs' total unmet facility needs. The section also requires the GAO to study the methodologies used by IHS in developing the health care facility priority system and in making facility needs assessments, and to report to specified committees of Congress and the Secretary. The section further requires the Secretary to consult with ITs and TOs, and confer with UIOs in developing innovative approaches to address unmet facility needs; and makes facility funds appropriated under the Snyder Act subject to ISDEAA.

Section 142. Priority of Certain Projects Protected

This section amends **IHCIA Section 301** [25 U.S.C. §1631] to add a new subsection that prohibits a project's priority in effect at enactment from being affected by a new facility priority system (see "Section 141. Health Care Facilities Priority System" above) if the project was identified in the FY2008 IHS budget justification as being in the top 10 for the four specified types of facilities; had completed both Phase I and Phase II of the construction priority system in effect prior to enactment; or is selected by the Secretary on the Secretary's initiative or pursuant to an IT or TO request.

Section 143. Indian Health Care Delivery Demonstration Project

This section amends **IHCIA Section 307** [25 U.S.C. §1637] by inserting new language that authorizes the Secretary to make grants to, or construction contracts or agreements with, ITs and TOs under ISDEAA to establish demonstration projects to test alternative health care delivery systems through health facilities to Indians, including through construction and renovation of hospitals, health centers, health stations, and other facilities or through cooperative agreements or other arrangements with other health care providers. The section specifies the uses of funds and permits their use to match federal and other funds. The section requires that equal criteria be used in evaluating tribal and IHS facilities, and requires integration of ISDEAA facility planning and construction into demonstration projects. The section defines "convenient care services" as any primary care service that is offered in an alternative setting or outside of regular working hours. The section also authorizes the Secretary to permit demonstration projects meeting certain specified criteria and gives preference to demonstration projects that meet these criteria and are located in the following Service Units: Cass Lake, MN; Mescaleroa, NM; Owyhee and Elko, NV; Schurz, NV; and Ft. Yuma, CA.

The Indian Health Care Improvement Act Reauthorization ... 113

In addition, the section requires the Secretary to promulgate regulations for application approval; it also establishes granting criteria, the grant selection process, and the requirements for technical assistance. The section also permits facilities, under the demonstration projects, to provide services to otherwise ineligible persons—that is, those who are not eligible for IHS services—and extends hospital privileges in IHS facilities to non-IHS health practitioners.

Section 144. Tribal Management of Federally Owned Quarters

This section adds a new **IHCIA Section 309** *Tribal Management of Federally Owned Quarters* [25 U.S.C. §1638a], which authorizes THPs operating a health care facility and the associated federally owned quarters pursuant to an ISDEAA contract or compact to establish reasonable rental rates for the federally owned quarters, by notifying the Secretary, and to collect the rent directly. The section sets the objectives of the THP's rental rates, requires that such quarters remain eligible for improvement and repair funds to the same extent as federally owned quarters, and requires at least 60 days' notice before changes in the rental rate. In addition, the section specifies requirements for direct rent collection by a THP, requires federal employees subject to the rent to pay the THP directly, and sets the effective date for a retrocession of rent collection authority. The provision also permits rental rates in Alaska to be comparable to those in the nearest established community with a year-round population of 1,500.

Section 145. Other Funding for Facilities

This section adds a new **IHCIA Section 311** *Other Funding, Equipment, and Supplies for Facilities* [25 U.S.C. §1638e], which authorizes the head of any federal agency that funds equipment or other supplies used for the planning, design, construction, or operation or a health care or sanitation facility (as defined) to transfer funds, equipment, or supplies to the Secretary. These transfers must be used for the planning, design, or construction of a health care or sanitation facility in accordance with the IHCIA, and with the purposes for which the funds were made available to the transferring agency. The section also authorizes the Secretary to accept such funds and use equipment and supplies for the planning, design, construction, and operation of health care and sanitation facilities for Indians, including facilities operated under ISDEAA contracts or compacts. In addition, the section states that funds received under this section must not affect facility priority established under IHCIA Section 301.

The section also authorizes the Secretary to enter into interagency agreements with federal or state agencies or other entities to accept funds, equipment, or supplies to plan, design, and construct health care or sanitation facilities to be administered by an IHP in order to carry out the purposes of IHCIA or the purposes for which the funds were appropriated or provided. The section requires the Secretary, acting through IHS, to establish, by regulation, standards for the planning design, construction, and operation of health care or sanitation facilities serving Indians under IHCIA; and requires that, notwithstanding other provisions of law, other applicable HHS regulations apply to funds transferred under this section.

Section 146. Modular Component Facilities Demonstration Program

This section adds a new **IHCIA Section 312** *Indian Country Modular Component Facilities Demonstration Program* [25 U.S.C. §1638f], which requires the Secretary, acting through the IHS, to establish a demonstration program to award grants for the establishment of not less than three modular component health care facilities (as defined). Grants will be awarded for the purchase, installation, and maintenance of such facilities in Indian communities for the provision of health care services. The section requires the Secretary to solicit petitions from ITs for modular component health care facilities; establishes petition criteria; and specifies that the Secretary is required to give priority to projects already on the IHS facilities construction priority list and to applications that demonstrate that modular facilities can be constructed more quickly and more economically than traditional facilities while adequately meeting health care service needs. The section also specifies that entities receiving grants under this section are not eligible for entry on the facilities construction priority list in FY2011 or any successor lists. ITs are eligible for grants under this section regardless of their participation in ISDEAA contracts or compacts. ITs and TOs receiving funds under this section are subject to ISDEAA. This section also requires the Secretary to submit a report, not later than one year after grants are awarded, describing grant activities and potential benefits. Finally, the section authorizes $50 million to be appropriated for the first five fiscal years and such sums as may be necessary in subsequent fiscal years.

Section 147. Mobile Health Stations Demonstration Program

This section adds a new **IHCIA Section 313** *Mobile Health Demonstration Program* [25 U.S.C. §1638g], which requires the Secretary, acting through the IHS, to establish a demonstration project to award funds for

The Indian Health Care Improvement Act Reauthorization ...   115

uses specified, including providing specialty health care (as defined) to at least three mobile health station projects (as defined by this section). Tribal consortia (as defined) are eligible for grants under this section after submitting a petition to the Secretary with required information. The Secretary is also required to submit a report to Congress, not later than one year after the demonstration has been established, describing and evaluating the demonstration program's activities and benefits. There are authorized to be appropriated $5 million for each of the first five fiscal years and such sums as may be necessary for each fiscal year thereafter to carry out the grant program under this section.

Subtitle D—Access to Health Services

Subtitle D amends IHCIA's Title IV "Access to Health Services," which authorizes IHS health care facilities to receive reimbursements from Social Security Act's (SSA's) Medicare and Medicaid programs. This authorization was a major component of the original IHCIA passed in 1976. The title establishes a "special fund" to receive the reimbursements and specifies what they can be used for. These reimbursements are an important source of funds for IHS. In FY2014, IHS estimated that it will receive approximately $1.1 billion from reimbursements.[34] These reimbursements are used to augment services received at IHS-funded facilities because IHCIA excludes Medicare or Medicaid reimbursements from being considered when determining annual Indian health appropriations. Other non-IHCIA sections of the ACA also make changes to IHSfunded facilities' ability to bill SSA programs and include provisions to increase American Indian and Alaska Native enrollment in these programs.

The ACA adds the State Children's Health Insurance Program (CHIP) to the programs that IHS health care facilities may bill, and expands the ability of THPs to bill these programs directly. In addition to amendments related to SSA programs, this subtitle also includes sections related to private insurance and sections related to coordination between IHS, the Department of Veterans Affairs (VA), and the Department of Defense (DOD).

Section 151. Treatment of Payments under SSA Health Benefits Programs

This section amends **IHCIA Section 401** [25 U.S.C. §1641] to require that payments received by an IHP or a UIO from Medicare, Medicaid, or

CHIP may not be considered in determining appropriations for Indian health care services. The section prohibits the Secretary from providing services to Indians with coverage under Medicare, Medicaid, or CHIP in preference to those Indians without such coverage. The section also requires that Medicare and Medicaid payments to IHS facilities be placed in a special fund held by the Secretary, and requires the Secretary to ensure that each IHS service unit receives 100% of the reimbursed amounts to which the service unit's facilities are entitled.

The section requires that amounts in the special fund be used by a facility first (to the extent provided in appropriations acts) to improve IHS facilities so they can comply with the applicable conditions and requirements of Medicare or Medicaid; if the reimbursed amounts are in excess of the amount necessary to make such improvements, the facilities are required to use the funds— after consulting with the tribes being served by the service unit—to reduce health resource deficiencies of Indian tribes, including for additional services authorized in IHCIA Section 205 ("Section 124. Other Authority for Provision of Services and Long-Term Care").

In addition, the section excludes THPs electing to receive payments directly from Medicare or Medicaid—called direct billing—from making payments into, or receiving from, the special fund. The section authorizes a THP to elect to directly bill and receive payments from Medicare, Medicaid, CHIP, or other third-party payors. The section requires that payments be used to improve THP facilities so they can comply with the applicable conditions and requirements of Medicare, Medicaid, or CHIP; or that payments be used to provide additional health care services, or to otherwise achieve the objectives in IHCIA Section 3 ("Section 103. Declaration of National Indian Health Policy"). The section also subjects THP direct payments to all auditing requirements applicable to whichever programs it chooses to bill directly and to all auditing requirements applicable to the IHP. The section requires that a THP receiving reimbursements or payments under Medicare, Medicaid, or CHIP provide to IHS a list of each provider enrollment number (or other identifier) under which the THP receives such reimbursements or payments and requires that IHS share this and other necessary information with the Centers for Medicare & Medicaid Services (CMS), the agency that administers the Medicare, Medicaid, and CHIP programs. The section also requires the Secretary, with assistance from CMS, to examine and implement any administrative changes that facilitate direct billing and reimbursement, including agreements with states necessary to provide for direct billing under Medicaid or CHIP. The section also permits participants (i.e., THPs) to

The Indian Health Care Improvement Act Reauthorization ... 117

withdraw from the program under the same conditions that an IT or TO may retrocede a contracted program under ISDEAA. In addition, the section authorizes the Secretary to terminate a direct billing participant if the Secretary determines that the participant has failed to comply with certain specified requirements, but requires the Secretary to provide notice and an opportunity to correct the noncompliance. The section cross-references specified sections of the SSA relating to the special fund and the direct billing program.

Section 152. Purchasing Health Care Coverage

This section amends **IHCIA Section 402** [25 U.S.C. §1642] to authorize ITs, TOs, or UIOs to use funds made available for health benefits for IHS beneficiaries under SSA programs, the ISDEAA (except for funds under IHCIA Section 402), or other law (except for Section 404) to purchase health benefits coverage. This may include coverage for service within a contract health service delivery area (CHSDA)[35] or any portion of a CHSDA that would have otherwise been provided by CHS; coverage through a tribally owned and operated health care plan, a state or locally authorized or licensed health care plan, a health insurance provider or managed care organization, or a self-insured plan. The section permits that purchased coverage be based on the financial needs of the individual beneficiaries (as determined by the tribe(s) being served) and permits funds to be used to operate a self-insured plan.

Section 153. SSA Health Benefit Programs Outreach and Enrollment Grants

This section amends **IHCIA Section 404** [25 U.S.C. §1644] to require the Secretary to make grants or enter into contracts with ITs and TOs for programs on or near reservations, trust lands, including using electronics and telecommunications, to assist individual Indians to enroll in Medicare, Medicaid, and CHIP, and other health benefit programs, and pay premiums and cost sharing required by the programs.[36] Payment of premiums and cost sharing may be based on need as determined by the IT or TO. The section also requires the Secretary, acting through IHS, to place conditions as deemed necessary on the contracts and grants, including requirements to determine Indian Medicaid, Medicare, and CHIP populations, educate Indians about the programs' benefits, provide transportation, and develop and implement methods to improve Indian participation in the programs. The section also applies the enrollment, premium, and cost-sharing assistance program to UIOs for the populations they serve, and sets requirements for agreements with such

118 Elayne J. Heisler

organizations. The section also requires the Secretary, acting through CMS, to consult with states, IHS, ITs, TOs, and UIOs on developing and disseminating best practices to facilitate agreements between the states, ITs, TOs, and UIOs regarding enrollment and retention of Indians in Medicare, Medicaid, and CHIP. The section cross references SSA Section 1139 regarding agreements for collecting, preparing, and submitting applications for Medicaid and CHIP. The section also defines the terms "premium" and "cost sharing."

Section 154. Sharing Arrangements with Federal Agencies

This section amends **IHCIA Section 405** [25 U.S.C. §1645] to insert new language that authorizes the Secretary to enter into or expand arrangements for IHS, ITs, and TOs to share medical facilities and services with the VA[37] and the DOD, but requires consultation with affected tribes prior to finalizing an arrangement. The section prohibits the Secretary from taking any action under this section that impairs (1) an Indian's priority access to, or eligibility for, health care services provided through IHS; (2) a veteran's priority access to VA health care services; (3) the quality of IHS health care provided to an Indian; (4) the quality of VA or DOD health care; or (5) an Indian veteran's eligibility to receive VA health care. The section requires reimbursement to the IHS, ITs, or TOs by the VA or DOD where beneficiaries eligible for VA or DOD services receive care from the IHS, ITs, or TOs.[38] The section prohibits construing the section as creating any right of a non-Indian veteran to IHS health services.

Section 155. Eligible Indian Veteran Services

This section adds a new **IHCIA Section 407** *Eligible Indian Veteran Services* [25 U.S.C. §1647], which makes a congressional finding that collaborations between the Secretary and the VA for treatment of Indian veterans at IHS facilities and increased enrollment for VA services by Indian tribal veterans should both be encouraged to the maximum extent practicable. The section also reaffirms the goals of a 2003 memorandum of understanding between IHS and VA's Veterans Health Administration regarding VA-authorized treatment of eligible Indian veterans at IHS facilities. The section requires the Secretary to provide for payment for veteran-related, VA-authorized treatment under a local memorandum of understanding. The section requires the Secretary to establish guidelines for such payments to the VA, and prohibits use of funds appropriated for IHS facilities, CHS, or contract support costs to make such payments. The section also requires the Secretary to consult with affected tribes in negotiating local memoranda of understanding,

The Indian Health Care Improvement Act Reauthorization ...   119

and defines "eligible Indian veteran" and "local memorandum of understanding."

Section 156. Nondiscrimination under Federal Health Care Programs

This section adds a new **IHCIA Section 408** *Nondiscrimination Under Federal Health Care Programs in Qualifications for Reimbursement for Services* [25 U.S.C. §1647a], which requires federal health care programs to accept an entity operated by IHS, an IT, TO, or a UIO, as a provider eligible to receive payment for health care services furnished to an Indian on the same basis as other qualified providers, if the Indian entity meets generally applicable state or other requirements for providers. The section requires that any requirement that providers be licensed or recognized under state or local law be deemed to have been met by such an Indian entity if the entity meets all applicable standards for licensure, regardless of whether it obtains a license. In accordance with Section 221, the section requires that the licensure of health professionals employed at Indian entities not be taken into account when determining if a facility meets licensure standards if the health professional is licensed in another state. The section also prohibits IHS, IT, TOs, and providers at these facilities from receiving payment or reimbursement from a federal health care program if the facility or provider has been excluded for participation in a federal health program or if the facility or provider's state license has been suspended or revoked. The section defines the term "Federal health care program" and cross-references SSA Section 1139 relating to nondiscrimination against providers operated by IHS, an IT, TO, or UIO.

Section 157. Access to Federal Insurance

This section adds a new **IHCIA Section 409** *Access to Federal Insurance* [25 U.S.C. §1647b], which specifies that, notwithstanding the provisions of Title V, the United States Code, an executive order, or an administrative regulation, an IT or TO carrying out programs under ISDEAA or a UIO carrying out programs under IHCIA Title V is entitled to purchase coverage, rights, and benefits for their employees under the Federal Employees Health Benefits Program[39] or the Federal Employees Group Life Insurance program.[40] The section also states that any necessary employee deductions and agency contributions are to be currently deposited in the Employee's Fund applicable to each program.

Section 158. Exception for Excepted Benefits

This section adds a new **IHCIA Section 410** *General Exceptions* [25 U.S.C. §1647c], which directs that the requirements of the previous provisions of IHCIA Title IV of this act may not apply to certain excepted benefits (involving coverage solely for accidents or disability insurance and certain coverage offered as non-coordinated benefits) defined in Section 2791(c) of the Public Health Service Act (PHSA).

Section 159. Navajo Nation Medicaid Agency Feasibility Study

This section adds a new **IHCIA Section 411** *Navajo Nation Medicaid Agency Feasibility Study* [25 U.S.C. §1647d], which requires the Secretary to conduct a study to determine the feasibility of treating the Navajo Nation[41] as a state for Medicaid purposes, for Indians living within the Navajo Nation's boundaries. The provision requires the Secretary to consider the feasibility of certain options and to report the results of the study to specified committees of Congress not later than three years after enactment.

Subtitle E—Health Services for Urban Indians

Subtitle E amends IHCIA Title V, which includes sections related to UIOs and services for urban Indians. Although IHS provides services primarily to American Indians and Alaska Natives living on or near reservations, more than half of this population resides in urban areas.[42] Programs funded under IHCIA Title V seek to make IHS more accessible and available to urban Indians.

There are 34 Urban Indian Health Programs (UIHPs). UIHPs may serve a wider range of eligible persons than the general IHS health care programs, such as members of terminated or state-recognized tribes and their children and grandchildren. These 34 UIHPs operate at 41 locations, with different programs offering different services, such as ambulatory health care, health promotion and education, immunizations, case management, and behavioral health services.[43] In addition to IHS grants and contracts, UIHPs receive funding from state and private sources, patient fees,[44] Medicaid, Medicare, and other non-IHS federal programs.[45]

The ACA maintains and amends existing IHCIA Title V sections and includes new sections that, for example, create new requirements for the Secretary to confer with UIOs, authorize the use of Community Health Representatives program (see IHCIA Title I, Section 109), and expand access to health information technology (HIT).

The Indian Health Care Improvement Act Reauthorization ...   121

Section 161. Facilities Renovation

This section amends **IHCIA Section 509** [25 U.S.C. §1659] to permit funds authorized under this section to be used by UIOs for the construction and expansion of facilities. Previously, funds authorized under this section could only be used to make minor renovations to facilities to meet or maintain the standards of the Joint Commission for Accreditation of Health Care Organizations (JCAHO).[46]

Section 162. Treatment of Certain Demonstration Projects

This section amends **IHCIA Section 513** [25 U.S.C. §1660c] to require that the Oklahoma City and Tulsa demonstration projects in Oklahoma (1) be permanent programs within IHS's direct care program; (2) continue to be treated as IHS service units and operating units in the allocation of resources and coordination of care; (3) continue to meet the requirements and definitions of UIOs under this act; and (4) not be subject to ISDEAA.

Section 163. Requirements to Confer with Urban Indian Organizations

This section adds a new **IHCIA Section 514** *Conferring with Urban Indian Organizations* [25 U.S.C. §1660d], which requires the Secretary to ensure that IHS confers or conferences with UIOs to the greatest extent practicable. It defines "confer" and "conference."

This section also amends **IHCIA Section 502** [25 U.S.C. §1652] to require the Secretary, under authority of the Snyder Act, to enter into contracts with or make grants to UIOs to establish in urban centers programs that meet the requirements of IHCIA Title V. In addition, the section requires the Secretary, acting through IHS and subject to IHCIA Section 506, to include within grants and contracts any conditions necessary to effect the purpose of IHCIA Title V.

Section 164. Expanded Program Authority for Urban Indian Organizations

This section adds a new **IHCIA Section 515** *Expanded Program Authority for Urban Indian Organizations* [25 U.S.C. §1660e] to authorize the Secretary, acting through IHS, to establish programs, including grants, for UIOs that are identical to programs established pursuant to IHCIA Section 218 (prevention of communicable diseases), Section 702 (behavioral health prevention and treatment services), and Section 708(g) (youth multidrug abuse program).

Section 165. Community Health Representatives

This section adds a new **IHCIA Section 516** *Community Health Representatives* [25 U.S.C. §1660f], which authorizes the Secretary to contract with or make grants to UIOs for the employment of Indians trained as health service providers through the Community Health Representatives Program under IHCIA Section 109.

Section 166. Use of Federal Government Facilities and Sources of Supply; HIT

This section adds a new **IHCIA Section 517** *Use of Federal Government Facilities and Sources of Supply* [25 U.S.C. §1660g], which authorizes the Secretary to (1) permit UIOs carrying out contracts or grants under this title to use existing HHS facilities and equipment; (2) donate excess IHS or General Services Administration real or personal property to such organizations; and (3) acquire excess or surplus federal government real or personal property for donation to such organizations (subject to a priority for tribes and tribal organizations). The section permits UIOs carrying out contracts or grants under this title to be deemed to be federal executive agencies under Section 201 of the Federal Property and Administrative Services Act of 1949, with access to federal prime vendors, when the organizations are carrying out IHCIA Title V contracts or grants.

This section also adds a new **IHCIA Section 518** *Health Information Technology* [25 U.S.C. §1660h], which authorizes the Secretary to make grants to UIOs under this title for the development, adoption, and implementation of HIT (as defined in PHSA Section 3000, telemedicine services development, and related infrastructure).

Subtitle F—Organizational Improvements

Subtitle F amends IHCIA Title VI. The title established IHS's organizational position as part of the PHS within HHS. The ACA reaffirms IHS's position in the PHS and establishes that the Director of IHS reports directly to the Secretary. The ACA also establishes an Office of Direct Service Tribes within IHS to address the needs of tribes that receive services administered by IHS as opposed to services administered by an IT or a TO under contract or compact (these are called direct service tribes). In addition, the ACA requires a plan for a new area office for tribes located in Nevada.

The Indian Health Care Improvement Act Reauthorization ...

Under the current IHS organization, tribes in Nevada receive services through the Phoenix Area Office.

Section 171. Establishment of the IHS as an Agency of the Public Health Service

This section amends **IHCIA Section 601** [25 U.S.C. §1661]. It maintains IHS's position within the Public Health Service, and maintains language establishing the IHS Director as an official appointed by the President with the advice and consent of the Senate for a four-year term. This section also amends IHCIA Section 601 to state that the IHS Director reports to the Secretary and the incumbent at enactment will remain as Director. The section specifies that the position of the Director reports directly to the Secretary on all policy and budget matters related to Indian health, interacts with assistant secretaries and agency heads on Indian health, and coordinates department activities on Indian health. The section maintains Indian preference for IHS employment.

Section 172. Office of Direct Service Tribes

This section adds a new **IHCIA Section 603** *Office of Direct Service Tribes* [25 U.S.C. §1663], which establishes an Office of Direct Service Tribes within the office of the IHS Director. The section also specifies the responsibilities of the new office, including providing leadership, guidance and support within IHS for direct service tribes, specified consultation responsibilities, and others.

Section 173. Nevada Area Office

This section adds a new **IHCIA Section 604** *Nevada Area Office* [25 U.S.C. §1663a], which requires the Secretary, in a manner consistent with IHS consultation policy, to submit to Congress, within one year of enactment, a plan to create a new Nevada Area Office distinct from the current Phoenix Area Office. If the Secretary fails to submit a plan, then the Secretary is required to withhold operation funds (as defined) from the IHS Office of the Director provided that such withholding does not adversely impact IHS health services. Withheld funds could be restored at the discretion of the Secretary when the plan is submitted.

Subtitle G—Behavioral Health Programs

Subtitle G amends IHCIA Title VII "Behavioral Health Programs," which includes sections that authorize behavioral health care programs. The ACA replaced the existing Title VII with new language that authorizes programs to create a "comprehensive behavioral health prevention and treatment program" providing a "continuum of behavioral health care" (see IHCIA Sections 701 and 703 of Section 181 below). The ACA also creates a new subsection of Title VII that authorizes new programs focused on preventing youth suicide.

Section 181. Behavioral Health Programs
This section replaces IHCIA Title VII with the following new programs:

Subtitle A—General Programs

Section 701. Definitions
This section adds a new **Section 701** *Definitions* [25 U.S.C. §1665], which defines a number of terms used in the title, including "Alcohol-related neurodevelopmental disorders," "dual diagnosis," "FAS or fetal alcohol syndrome," "rehabilitation," and "substance abuse."

Section 702. Behavioral Health Prevention and Treatment Services
This section adds a new **Section 702** *Behavioral Health Prevention and Treatment Service* [25 U.S.C. §1665a]. The section includes the purpose of the title, which includes directing the Secretary, acting through IHS, to develop a comprehensive behavioral health care program that emphasizes collaboration among alcohol and substance abuse, social services, and mental health programs. The section also requires the Secretary to encourage ITs, TOs, and UIOs to develop tribal, local, and area-wide plans for Indian behavioral health services that include assessments of specified behavioral problems, the number of Indians affected, the financial and human costs, the existing and necessary resources to prevent and treat such problems, and an estimate of necessary funding. The section requires the Secretary to coordinate with existing national clearinghouses to include such plans and any reports on their outcomes; ensure access to the plans and outcomes by IHS, ITs, TOs, and UIOs; and provide technical assistance in the development of these plans and related standards of care. The section also requires the Secretary to provide, through IHS, and to the extent feasible and funded, a comprehensive continuum of behavioral health care, as well as specified services for Indian children, adults, families,

The Indian Health Care Improvement Act Reauthorization ...   125

and elders. The section authorizes ITs, TOs, and UIOs to establish community behavioral health plans, requires IHS and BIA cooperation and assistance in developing and implementing such plans, and authorizes grants to ITs and TOs for technical assistance and administrative support for such plans. The section requires the Secretary, through IHS, ITs, TOs, and UIOs, to coordinate behavioral health planning with other federal and state agencies. The section also requires the Secretary, within one year of enactment, to assess the need, availability, and cost for inpatient mental health care and facilities for Indians, including possible conversion of existing, underused IHS hospital beds into psychiatric units.

Section 703. Memoranda of Agreement with the Department of Interior

This section adds a new **IHCIA Section 703** *Memoranda of Agreement with the Department of Interior*[47] [25 U.S.C. §1665b], which requires the Secretary and the Secretary of the Interior, not later than 12 months after enactment, to develop and enter into memoranda of agreement, or update the memoranda of agreement required by Section 4205 of the Indian Alcohol and Substance Abuse Prevention and Treatment Act.[48] The section specifies that the memoranda of agreement must address eight specified activities, including a comprehensive assessment and coordination of mental health care needs and services available or unavailable to Indians, and the ensuring and protection of Indians' right of access to general mental health services. The section further requires that the memoranda include provisions assigning to IHS responsibility for determining the scope of alcohol and substance abuse problems among Indians, assessing existing and needed resources, and estimating necessary funding. The section also requires that each memorandum, renewal, or modification be published in the *Federal Register*, with copies to ITs, TOs, and UIOs.

Section 704. Behavioral Health Prevention and Treatment Program

This section adds a new **Section 704** *Comprehensive Behavioral Health Prevention and Treatment Program* [25 U.S.C. §1665c], which requires the Secretary to provide, through IHS, a program of comprehensive behavioral health, prevention, treatment, and aftercare, for Indian tribal members that includes education, specified treatments, rehabilitation, training, and diagnostic services. The section authorizes the Secretary, through IHS, to provide the services through contracts with public and private behavioral health providers, and requires the Secretary to assist ITs and TOs with developing criteria for certification of providers and accreditation of facilities.

Section 705. Mental Health Technician Program

This section adds a new **Section 705** *Mental Health Technician Program* [25 U.S.C. §1665d], which requires the Secretary, under the Snyder Act, to establish within IHS a mental health technician training and employment program for Indians. The section also requires the Secretary, through IHS, to provide high-standard paraprofessional training in mental health care, to supervise and evaluate these technicians, and to ensure that the program includes using and promoting traditional Indian health care practices of the tribes served.

Section 706. Licensing Requirement for Mental Health Care Workers

This section adds a new **Section 706** *Licensing Requirement for Mental Health Care Workers* [25 U.S.C. §1665e], which, subject to IHCIA Section 221 (regarding licensing), requires that any person employed as a psychologist, social worker, or marriage and family therapist to provide mental health care services to Indians in a clinic be licensed to provide the specified service. The section also provides that a trainee in psychology, social work, or marriage and family therapy may provide mental health care services if the trainee is directly supervised by someone licensed in the specified service, is enrolled in or has completed at least two years of course work in an accredited post-secondary education program for the specified service, and meets other requirements that the Secretary may establish.

Section 707. Indian Women Treatment Programs

This section adds a new **Section 707** *Indian Women Treatment Programs* [25 U.S.C. §1665f], which authorizes the Secretary, consistent with IHCIA Section 701, to make grants to ITs, TOs, and UIOs to develop and implement a comprehensive behavioral health program for prevention, intervention, treatment, and relapse prevention that specifically addresses the cultural, historical, social, and childcare needs of Indian women. The section specifies uses of the grants, including community training and education, counseling, support, and development of prevention and intervention models. The section also requires the Secretary, in consultation with ITs and TOs, to establish grant approval criteria, and to allocate 20% of the program's funds for grants to UIOs.

Section 708. Indian Youth Program

This section adds a new **Section 708** *Indian Youth Program* [25 U.S.C. §1665g], which establishes a number of Indian youth behavioral health

The Indian Health Care Improvement Act Reauthorization ...   127

programs. The section requires the Secretary, consistent with IHCIA Section 701, to develop and implement a program for acute detoxification and treatment for Indian youth, including behavioral health services, regional treatment centers with detoxification and rehabilitation services, and local programs developed by ITs or TOs under ISDEAA. The section requires the Secretary, through IHS, to construct, renovate, or purchase, and staff and operate (under the Snyder Act) at least one youth regional treatment center or treatment network in each IHS area (treating the California Area as two areas), in a location agreed upon by a majority of the area's tribes; the section also authorizes funding to two specified Alaska Native entities for youth treatment facilities in Alaska.[49] The section authorizes the Secretary to provide intermediate behavioral health services for Indian children and adolescents, and specifies that such services include pretreatment assistance; inpatient, outpatient, and aftercare services; emergency care; suicide prevention; and prevention and treatment of mental illness and dysfunctional and self-destructive behavior, including child abuse and family violence. The section sets the allowable uses of funds for intermediate behavioral health services, and requires the Secretary, in consultation with ITs and TOs, to develop grant approval criteria.

The section also requires the Secretary, in consultation with ITs and TOs, to identify and use suitable federally owned structures for local residential or regional behavioral health treatment for Indian youths, and establish suitability guidelines. The section allows the use of any such federally owned structure under terms agreed upon by the Secretary, the responsible federal agency, and the IT or TO operating the program. The section also requires the Secretary, ITs, and TOs, in cooperation with the Secretary of Interior, to develop local community-based rehabilitation and aftercare services provided by trained staff in each IHS service unit for Indian youths with significant behavioral health problems, including long-term treatment, community reintegration, and monitoring. The section requires the Secretary, in providing services under this section, to provide for inclusion of family in such services, and specifies that not less than 10% of funds for the local rehabilitation and aftercare services program may be used for outpatient care of adult family members of an Indian youth in the program. The section also requires the Secretary, through IHS, to provide programs and services to prevent and treat multi-drug abuse among Indian youths in Indian communities, on or near reservations, and in urban areas, and provide appropriate mental health services. The section requires the Secretary to collect data on specified aspects of Indian youth mental health for the report under IHCIA Section 801.

Section 709. Mental Health Facilities Design, Construction, and Staffing

This section adds a new **Section 709** *Inpatient and Community-Based Mental Health Facilities Design, Construction, and Staffing* [25 U.S.C. §1665h], which authorizes the Secretary, through IHS, to provide in each IHS area, not later than one year after enactment, at least one inpatient mental health facility for Indians with behavioral health problems. The section requires that California be considered two areas and requires the Secretary to consider the conversion of existing underused IHS hospital beds into psychiatric units to meet the need for such facilities.

Section 710. Training and Community Education

This section adds a new **Section 710** *Training and Community Education* [25 U.S.C. §1665i], which requires the Secretary, in cooperation with the Secretary of the Interior, to develop and implement in each IHS service unit or tribal program a program of community education and involvement for specified tribal community leaders in behavioral health issues, possibly including community-based training, or to assist tribes and tribal organizations in doing so. The section requires the Secretary to provide specified instruction in behavioral health issues to appropriate IHS and BIA employees and personnel in contracted IHS and BIA programs and schools.[50] In addition, this section requires the Secretary, as part of the community education and employee instruction programs, to develop and provide community-based training models addressing specified aspects of behavioral health problems, in consultation with ITs, TOs, and Indian alcohol and substance abuse prevention experts.

Section 711. Behavioral Health Program

This section adds a new **Section 711** *Behavioral Health Program* [25 U.S.C. §1665j], which authorizes the Secretary, through IHS, to develop and implement programs to deliver innovative community-based behavioral health services to Indians, and authorize grants to ITs and TOs for such programs. The section specifies criteria for awarding such grants, and requires the Secretary to use the same criteria in evaluating all project applications.

Section 712. Fetal Alcohol Spectrum Disorder Programs

This section adds a new **Section 712** *Fetal Alcohol Spectrum Disorders Programs* [25 U.S.C. §1665k], which authorizes the Secretary, through IHS, to develop and implement fetal alcohol disorder (FAD) programs (as defined in IHCIA Section 4), consistent with IHCIA Section 701, and to establish criteria

The Indian Health Care Improvement Act Reauthorization ...   129

for approval of funding applications. The section specifies grant uses, including developing and providing services for the prevention, intervention, treatment, and aftercare for those affected by FAD; early childhood intervention projects; supportive services; and housing. The section requires the Secretary, through IHS, to provide FAD prevention, treatment, and aftercare services as well as specified support services.

The section also requires the Secretary to make grants through the Substance Abuse and Mental Health Services Administration (SAMHSA) in HHS to ITs, TOs, and UIOs for applied research projects to elevate the understanding of methods to prevent, intervene, treat, or provide rehabilitation and aftercare for Indians affected by fetal alcohol spectrum disorders. The section requires that 10% of appropriations under this section be used for grants to UIOs funded under IHCIA Title V.

Section 713. Child Sexual Abuse Prevention and Treatment Programs

This section adds a new **Section 713** *Child Sexual Abuse Prevention and Treatment Programs* [25 U.S.C. §1665l], which requires the Secretary, through IHS, and consistent with IHCIA Section 701, to establish in every IHS Area treatment programs for child victims of sexual abuse who are Indians or members of Indian households. The section requires four uses of funding, including developing community education, identifying and providing treatment to victims, and developing culturally sensitive prevention models and diagnostic tools. The section requires that the programs be carried out in coordination with programs and services authorized under the Indian Child Protection and Family Violence Prevention Act.[51]

Section 714. Domestic and Sexual Violence Prevention and Treatment

This section adds a new **Section 714** *Domestic and Sexual Violence Prevention and Treatment* [25 U.S.C. §1665m], which authorizes the Secretary to establish programs in each IHS Area to prevent and treat Indian victims of domestic violence or sexual violence. The section requires that program funds be used for prevention and community education programs, behavioral health services and medical treatment for victims (including examinations by sexual assault nurse examiners), rape kits, and development of prevention and intervention models (including traditional health care). The section requires the Secretary to establish protocols, policies, procedures, standards, training curricula, and training and certification requirements for victim services within one year of enactment, and requires a report on these activities to specified committees of Congress within 18 months of enactment.

The section also requires the Secretary, in coordination with the Attorney General (AG), federal and tribal law enforcement agencies, IHPs, and victim organizations, to develop victim services and victim advocate training programs, for specified purposes, and it requires the Secretary, within two years of enactment, to report to specified committees of Congress on such services and programs, including improvements, obstacles, costs needed to address the obstacles, and any recommendations.

Section 715. Behavioral Health Research

This section adds a new **Section 715** *Behavioral Health Research* [25 U.S.C. §1665n], which requires the Secretary, in consultation with appropriate federal agencies, to make contracts with or grants to ITs, TOs, and UIOs, and appropriate institutions for research on the incidence and prevalence of behavioral health problems among Indians served by IHS, ITs, or TOs and in urban areas. The section directs that research priorities include the multifactorial causes of Indian youth suicide; the interrelationship of behavioral health problems with alcoholism, suicide, homicide, and family violence, especially on children; and the development of models of prevention techniques, especially in regard to children.

Subtitle B—Indian Youth Suicide Services

Section 721. Findings and Purpose

This section adds a new **Section 721** *Findings and Purpose* [25 U.S.C. §1667], which includes the findings and the stated purposes of this section, which are (1) to authorize the Secretary to carry out a demonstration project to test the use of telemental health services in suicide prevention, intervention, and treatment of Indian youth (through specified means); (2) to encourage ITs, TOs, and other mental health care providers serving residents of Indian country to obtain the services of predoctoral psychology and psychiatry interns; and (3) to enhance the provision of mental health care services to Indian youth through existing SAMHSA grants.

Section 722. Definitions

This section adds a new **Section 722** *Definitions* [25 U.S.C. §1667a], which defines the following terms: "Administration," "demonstration project," and "telemental health."

Section 723. Indian Youth Telemental Health Demonstration Project

This section adds a new **Section 723** *Indian Youth Telemental Health Demonstration Project* [25 U.S.C. §1667b], which authorizes the Secretary to carry out a demonstration project by making four-year grants to not more than five ITs and TOs with telehealth capabilities to use for telemental health services in youth suicide prevention and treatment. The section defines terms and directs the Secretary to give priority to ITs and TOs that serve tribal communities that have a demonstrated need or are isolated and have limited access to mental health services, that enter into collaborative partnerships to provide the services, or that operate a detention facility where youth are detained. The section describes the uses of the grants, including the use of telemedicine for psychotherapy, psychiatric assessments, and diagnostic interviews of Indian youth; the provision of clinical expertise and other medical advice to frontline health care providers working with Indian youth; training and related support for community leaders, family members, and health and education workers who work with Indian youth; the development of culturally relevant educational materials on suicide prevention and intervention; data collection and reporting; and the use of the tribe's traditional health care practices. The section includes requirements for grant applications, encourages collaboration among grantees and grantee reports to the national clearinghouse under IHCIA Section 701, and requires grantees to submit annual reports to the Secretary. In addition, the section requires the Secretary to submit a report to specified committees of Congress no later than 270 days after termination of the demonstration project. The report must include evaluations of whether the project should be made permanent or expanded to more than five grants and to UIOs. The section authorizes appropriations of such sums as may be necessary to carry out this section.

Section 724. SAMHSA Grants

This section adds a new **Section 724** *Substance Abuse and Mental Health Services Administration Grants* [25 U.S.C. §1667c], which requires the Secretary to streamline the process by which ITs and TOs could apply for SAMHSA grants, including providing non-electronic methods. For SAMHSA grants for activities relating to mental health, suicide prevention, or suicide-related risk factors, and for which an IT or TO is eligible, in order to fulfill the trust responsibility of the United States to ITs, the Secretary is required to consider the needs of ITs or TOs that serve populations with documented high suicide rates, regardless of whether those ITs or TOs possess adequate personnel or infrastructure to fulfill all applicable grant requirements.

Notwithstanding any other provision of law, no IT or TO is required to apply for SAMHSA grants through a state or state agency. Any state applying for a SAMHSA grant based on statewide data is required to consider the Indian population within the state and make reasonable efforts to collaborate with ITs within the state in implementing SAMHSA grant programs. ITs and TOs are not required to provide non-federal contributions for any SAMHSA grant. The Secretary is also required to conduct outreach to rural and isolated tribes to promote the purposes of this subtitle. The Secretary is required to take other measures to assure access to mental health and suicide prevention services by ITs at high risk, as defined by suicide rates, socioeconomic status, and other factors. The section also authorizes to be appropriated such sums as may be necessary to carry out this section. Finally, the Secretary is required to ensure that any recipient of a grant under PHSA Section 520E (grants for youth suicide prevention and early intervention strategies that are not exclusive to tribal awardees) provides training to those serving Indian youth under the grant program in the recognition of suicide risk among Indian youth.

Section 725 Use of Predoctoral Psychology and Psychiatry Interns

This section adds a new **Section 725** *Use of Predoctoral Psychology and Psychiatry Interns* [25 U.S.C. §1667d], which requires the Secretary to carry out activities to encourage ITs, TOs, and other mental health care providers to obtain the services of predoctoral psychology and psychiatry interns in order to increase the quantity of patients served by those providers, and for purposes of recruitment and retention.

Section 726. Indian Youth Life Skills Demonstration Program

This section adds a new **Section 726** *Indian Youth Life Skills Development Demonstration Program* [25 U.S.C. §1667e], which authorizes the Secretary, through SAMHSA, to carry out a demonstration program to test the effectiveness of a culturally compatible, school-based, life skills curriculum for the prevention of American Indian and Alaska Native adolescent suicide. The program may use tribal partnerships, assistance from SAMHSA, training, advisory councils, and other approaches. The section also authorizes the Secretary to award demonstration grants to ITs, TOs, or other authorized entities or partnerships who meet specified application requirements, to implement the life skills curriculum. Not more than five grants may be awarded for terms of not less than four years, and at least one grant must be awarded to each of (1) a school operated by the Bureau of Indian Education (BIE); (2) a Tribal school; and (3) a school receiving payments under Section

The Indian Health Care Improvement Act Reauthorization ...   133

8002 or 8003 of the Elementary and Secondary Education Act of 1965. Grant funds may be used for a number of specific activities. The Secretary is also required to conduct annual program evaluations, and to report to Congress regarding the program within 180 days of its termination, following a public comment period. The section authorizes an appropriation of $1 million for each of FY2010 through FY2014.[52]

Subtitle H—Miscellaneous

Subtitle H amends IHCIA Title VIII, which includes a number of miscellaneous provisions, including those that require annual reports about activities authorized in IHCIA, and those related to a number of demonstration programs in specified topics and areas. The ACA amends existing sections about certain persons' eligibility for IHS services; adds new sections about medical records; the designation of CHSDAs; IHS budget submissions; monitoring of prescription drugs; required reports; and a variety of other topics.

Section 191. Medical Quality Assurance Records Confidentiality

This section adds a new **IHCIA Section 805** [25 U.S.C. §1675], which makes medical quality assurance records created by an IHP or a UIHP confidential and privileged, and prohibits their disclosure except to specified entities for specified purposes. The section exempts such records from the Freedom of Information Act,[53] requires the Secretary to promulgate regulations, and defines terms.

Section 192. Arizona, North Dakota, and South Dakota as CHSDAs

This section amends **IHCIA Section 808** [25 U.S.C. §1678] with a new section *Arizona as a Contract Health Service Delivery Area* that designates the state of Arizona as an IHS CHSDA for the members of ITs in Arizona. The section also prohibits IHS from curtailing any services as a result of this section.

This section also adds a new **IHCIA Section 808A** *North Dakota and South Dakota as CHSDAs* [25 U.S.C. §1678a], which designates North Dakota and South Dakota as one CHSDA for the purpose of providing CHS to members of ITs in these states. This section also prohibits IHS from curtailing any services as a result of this provision.

This section also amends **IHCIA Section 809** [25 U.S.C. §1679] with a new section *Eligibility of California Indians* that designates specified California Indians as eligible for IHS health services, including members of federally recognized tribes, descendants of Indians residing in California as of June 1, 1852 (if living in California and meeting other criteria), Indians holding trust interests in certain types of land, and Indians (and their descendants) listed on the plans for asset distribution in California under the Act of August 18, 1958 (terminating recognition of certain California tribes). The section prohibits construing anything in the section as expanding California Indians' eligibility for IHS health services beyond their eligibility as of May 1, 1986.

Section 193. Methods to Increase Access to Health Professionals

This section adds a new **IHCIA Section 812** *National Health Service Corps* [25 U.S.C. §1680b], which prohibits the Secretary from removing a member of the National Health Service Corps (NHSC)[54] from an IHP or UIO, or withdrawing funding to support such member, unless the Secretary, acting through the IHS, ensures that Indians will experience no reduction in services. The section also authorizes that, at the IHP's request, the services of NHSC personnel assigned to an IHP may be limited to the persons eligible for services from such program.

Section 194. Health Services for Ineligible Persons

This section amends **IHCIA Section 813** [25 U.S.C. §1680c] with new language that authorizes IHS health services for certain otherwise ineligible persons, including spouses or children of eligible Indians, non-Indian women carrying Indian babies, or persons in need of emergency stabilization, or for prevention of communicable diseases. The section authorizes the governing body of Indian tribes operating health facilities under ISDEAA contracts to determine whether to provide services to ineligible persons. The section also sets criteria for providing services, such as requiring reimbursement and tribal approval, and directs that reimbursements, including under Medicare or Medicaid, be credited to the facility providing the service and be available for expenditure by the facility. The section permits the Secretary to provide services to indigent individuals who are not otherwise eligible for IHS services provided that the state or local government agrees to reimburse IHS for providing this service. The section also permits extending hospital privileges to non-IHS health care practitioners who provide service to certain ineligible persons.

Section 195. Annual Budget Submission

This section adds a new **IHCIA Section 826** *Annual Budget Submission* [25 U.S.C. §1680p], which requires the President, effective with the submission of the FY2011 budget, to request amounts that reflect changes in the cost of health care services as adjusted by the consumer price index for inflation, and amounts that reflect changes in the size of the population served by IHS.

Section 196. Prescription Drug Monitoring

This sections adds a new **IHCIA Section 827** *Prescription Drug Monitoring* [25 U.S.C. §1680q], which requires the Secretary, in coordination with the Secretary of the Interior and AG, to establish a prescription drug monitoring program, to be carried out at facilities operated by IHS, ITs, TOs, and UIOs. The section also requires the Secretary to submit a report within 18 months of enactment to specified congressional committees describing (1) the prescription drug monitoring program needs of facilities operated by IHS, ITs, TOs, and UIOs; (2) the planned development and the means to carry out a prescription drug monitoring program, including relevant statutory or administrative limitations; and (3) the need for coordination with any state prescription drug monitoring program. The section requires the AG, in conjunction with the Secretary and the Secretary of the Interior, to conduct (1) an assessment of the capacity of, and support required by, relevant federal and tribal agencies to collect and analyze data and exchange information regarding incidents of prescription drug abuse in Indian communities and exchange information regarding prescription drug abuse in Indian communities; and (2) training for Indian health care providers, tribal leaders, law enforcement, and school officials regarding awareness and prevention of prescription drug abuse and strategies to improve and address prescription drug abuse in Indian communities. The section also requires the AG, within 18 months of enactment, to submit a report to specified congressional committees that describes certain factors regarding the AG's responsibilities related to prescription drug abuse in Indian communities.[55]

Section 197. Tribal Health Program Option for Cost Sharing

This section adds a new **IHCIA Section 828** *Tribal Health Program Option for Cost Sharing* [25 U.S.C. §1680r], which states that nothing in IHCIA limits the ability of a THP operating any health program, service, function, activity, or facility funded in whole or in part by IHS through a compact with IHS under Title V of the ISDEAA, to charge an Indian for services provided by the THP. The section also states that nothing in IHCIA authorizes IHS to charge an Indian for services or to require a THP to charge an Indian for services.

Section 198. Disease and Injury Prevention Reports

This section adds a new **IHCIA Section 829** *Disease and Injury Prevention* [25 U.S.C. §1680s], which requires the Secretary to submit, within 18 months of enactment, a report to specified congressional committees describing all disease and injury prevention activities conducted by IHS either independently or in conjunction with federal departments, agencies, and ITs, and the effectiveness of such activities.

Section 199. Other GAO Reports

This section adds new **IHCIA Section 830** *Other GAO Reports* [25 U.S.C. §1680t], which requires two specified GAO reports to be submitted to Congress within 18 months of enactment. GAO must conduct studies on (1) the effectiveness of the coordination of health care services provided to Indians: (a) through Medicare, Medicaid, or CHIP; (b) by IHS; or (c) by using funds provided by state or local governments or ITs; and (2) the use of CHS including analyses of amounts reimbursed to providers, suppliers, and entities under CHS, compared to reimbursements through other public and private programs; barriers to access to health care under CHS; adequacy of federal funding of CHS; and other matters GAO determines appropriate. This study must be conducted in consultation with IHS, ITs, and TOs, and must include recommendations on appropriate federal funding for CHS and ways to use such funding efficiently.[56]

Section 200. Traditional Health Care Practices

This section adds a new **IHCIA Section 831** *Traditional Health Care Practices* [25 U.S.C. §1680u], which states that the United States is not liable for damage, injuries, or death that may result from traditional health care practices, consistent with IHS standards for the provision of health care, health promotion, and disease prevention provided pursuant to IHCIA (although the Secretary may promote traditional health care practices). The section further specifies that nothing in the section may be construed to alter any liability of other obligation that the United States has under ISDEAA.

The Indian Health Care Improvement Act Reauthorization ...   137

Section 201. Director of HIV/AIDS Prevention and Treatment

This section adds a new **IHCIA Section 832** *Director of HIV/AIDS Prevention and Treatment* [25 U.S.C. §1680v], which requires the Secretary, acting through IHS, to establish within IHS a Director of HIV/AIDS Prevention and Treatment.

The Director is required to (1) coordinate and promote HIV/AIDS prevention and treatment activities for Indians; (2) provide technical assistance to ITs, TOs, and UIOs regarding existing HIV/AIDS prevention and treatment programs; and (3) ensure interagency coordination to facilitate the inclusion of Indians in federal HIV/AIDS research and grant opportunities with an emphasis on programs operated under the Ryan White Comprehensive AIDS Resource Emergency Act of 1990[57] and its amendments.

The section also requires that, not later than two years after enactment and every two years thereafter, the Director submit to Congress a report describing the activities carried out under this section and the Director's findings related to HIV/AIDS prevention and treatment activities specific to Indians.

Section 10221(b)(3) Abortion Funding Restrictions

This section amends **IHCIA Section 806** [25 U.S.C. §1676] to state that any funds appropriated to HHS may not be used for the performance or coverage of abortion.

In addition, the section states that any limitation included in another federal law with respect to the performance or coverage of abortion also applies to funds appropriated to IHS.

TITLE II—AMENDMENTS TO OTHER ACTS[58]

Title II of the Indian Health Care Improvement Reauthorization and Extension Act, as enacted, contains one provision that amends and reauthorizes the Native Hawaiian Health Care Act of 1988 (NHHCA, P.L. 100-579, as amended; 42 U.S.C. §11701-11714), which authorizes health education, health promotion, disease prevention services, and health professions scholarship programs for Native Hawaiians.[59]

Section 202. Reauthorization of Native Hawaiian Health Care Programs

This section reauthorizes expired appropriations authorities in the NHHCA [42 U.S.C. §11701- 11714] through FY2019. This section also amends the NHHCA [42 U.S.C. §11705], effective on December 5, 2006, to permit a specified private educational organization (Kamehameha Schools Bishop Estate) identified in Section 7202(16) of the Elementary and Secondary Education Act of 1965 [20 U.S.C.7512(16)] to continue to offer educational programs and services to Native Hawaiians (as defined in that act) first, and to other groups only after the needs of Native Hawaiians have been met. This section also amends the definition of "health promotion" in NHHCA Section 12(2).

APPENDIX A. TIMELINE OF IHCIA PROVISIONS IN THE ACA

In some instances, the ACA specifies dates for key administrative or programmatic activities or requirements. The following timeline (see **Table A-1**) lists the provisions summarized in this report that include dates, such as those that include dates for reports.

Other activities or requirements that have no date specified in the ACA and are implicitly effective upon enactment (March 23, 2010) are not included in this timeline. All activities authorized in the IHCIA are discretionary and subject to appropriations by Congress. Given this, all deadlines below may not be considered binding since they are subject to appropriated funds. Where available, the timeline includes information on action that IHS, or other federal agencies, have taken in response to deadlines within the two and a half years after enactment (i.e., through September 23, 2012).

Table A-1 lists the ACA dates, which are grouped by subtitle in the IHCIA Reauthorization and Extension Act of 2009. Not all subtitles are included, as some subtitles do not include provisions with specified deadlines. Within each subtitle, table entries are organized with key dates in chronological order.

Table A-1. Timeline of IHCIA Provisions in the ACA

Section of the IHCIA Reauthorization and Extension Act of 2009 as enacted by ACA Section 10221	Title	Description	Start or Effective Date or Deadline
Subtitle B–Health Services			
Section 127	Behavioral Training and Community Education Programs	Requires the Secretary to develop a plan to increase behavioral health services by creating 500 additional staff positions within 5 years of enactment.	6/21/2010
Section 133	Prevention and Control of Communicable Diseases	Requires the Secretary to submit a biennial report to Congress on the grants awarded for the prevention, control, and elimination of communicable and infectious diseases.	3/23/2012
Section 136	Office of Indian Men's Health	Requires the Secretary, through IHS, to submit a report to Congress describing the activities carried out by the Office of Indian Men's Health and findings related to Indian Men's Health.	3/23/2012
Section 121	Indian Health Care Improvement Fund	Requires the Secretary to submit a report to Congress on the current health status and resource deficiencies of each tribe or service unit.	3/23/2013

Section of the IHCIA Reauthorization and Extension Act of 2009 as enacted by ACA Section 10221	Title	Description	Start or Effective Date or Deadline
Section 137	CHS Administration and Disbursement Formula	Requires GAO to submit a report to Congress describing the results of a study about the CHS program including funding levels and administration of the program.	As soon as practicabl e after enactment
Subtitle C–Health Facilities			
Section 141	Health Care Facilities Priority System	Requires the Secretary, in the annual report required in Section 801, to submit a report to the President describing the health care facility priority system and the top 10 priorities for various construction projects under this priority system.	February 7, 2011a
Section 141	Health Care Facilities Priority System	Requires the Secretary to submit an initial report to Congress with a ranked list of all IHS, IT, and TO health care facility needs. Further requires the Secretary to submit an updated version of this report every 5 years beginning in 2011.	3/23/2011

Section of the IHCIA Reauthorization and Extension Act of 2009 as enacted by ACA Section 10221	Title	Description	Start or Effective Date or Deadline
Section 141	Health Care Facilities Priority System	Requires GAO to study the methodologies used by IHS to develop its health care priority system.	One year after new priority system is developed
Section 147	Mobile Health Station Demonstration Program	Requires the Secretary to submit a report to Congress that describes and evaluates the results of a demonstration project establishing mobile health stations.	One year after the demonstration program is established
Subtitle D–Access to Health Services			
Section 159	Navajo Nation Medicaid Agency Feasibility Study	Requires the Secretary to submit a report to Congress considering the feasibility of considering the Navajo Nation a state for Medicaid purposes.	3/23/2013
Subtitle F–Organizational Improvements			
Section 173	Nevada Area Office	Requires the Secretary to submit a plan to Congress to create a new Nevada Area Office.	3/23/2011
Subtitle G–Behavioral Health Programs			
Section 181 (Section 702)	Behavioral Health Prevention and Treatment Services	Requires the Secretary, acting through IHS, to assess the need, availability, and cost of inpatient mental health care for Indians.	3/23/2011

Section of the IHCIA Reauthorization and Extension Act of 2009 as enacted by ACA Section 10221	Title	Description	Start or Effective Date or Deadline
Section 181 (Section 703)	Memoranda of Agreement with the Department of the Interior	Requires the Secretary, acting through IHS, and the Secretary of the Interior to develop and enter into a memorandum of agreement regarding mental illness and self-destructive behavior among Indians and strategies to address unmet needs.	3/23/2011
Section 181 (Section 714)	Domestic and Sexual Violence Prevention and Treatment	Requires the Secretary to establish protocols, policies, procedures, and programs for victims of domestic or sexual violence.	3/23/2011
Section 181 (Section 714)	Domestic and Sexual Violence Prevention and Treatment	Requires the Secretary to submit a report to Congress on protocols, policies, procedures, and other programs for victims of domestic or sexual violence.	9/23/2011
Section 181 (Section 714)	Domestic and Sexual Violence Prevention and Treatment	Requires the Secretary to submit a report to Congress on domestic and sexual violence prevention and treatment programs. The report should also include improvement needed, obstacles faced, and costs of addressing these obstacles.	3/23/2012

Section of the IHCIA Reauthorization and Extension Act of 2009 as enacted by ACA Section 10221	Title	Description	Start or Effective Date or Deadline
Section 181 (Section 726)	Indian Youth Life Skills Demonstration Program	Requires the Secretary to report on the results of a program evaluation conducted on a demonstration program to test the effectiveness of programs to prevent American Indian and Alaska Native suicide.	180 days after the termination of the demonstration program and after the public comment period.
Subtitle H–Miscellaneous			
Section 195	Annual Budget Submission	Requires the President to include, within the IHS annual budget request and justification, amounts that reflect changes in the cost of health care services adjusted by the consumer price index and amounts adjusted to reflect changes in the IHS service population.	February 1, 2010b
Section 196	Prescription Drug Monitoring	Requires the Secretary to submit a report describing the specified elements of the prescription drug monitoring program.	9/23/2011

Section of the IHCIA Reauthorization and Extension Act of 2009 as enacted by ACA Section 10221	Title	Description	Start or Effective Date or Deadline
Section 196	Prescription Drug Monitoring	Requires the AG to submit a report to Congress describing certain factors regarding the AG's responsibility related to prescription drug abuse in Indian communities.	9/23/2011
Section 198	Disease and Injury Prevention Reports	Requires the Secretary to submit a report to Congress describing disease and injury prevention activities by IHS and other federal agencies.	9/23/2011
Section 199	Other GAO Reports	Requires GAO to submit a report to Congress containing the results and recommendations resulting from a study evaluating the effectiveness of the coordination of health care services provided to Indians either through Medicare, Medicaid, or CHIP, with those provided by IHS, with funding from state or local governments or ITs.	9/23/2011
Section 199	Other GAO Reports	Requires the Comptroller General to study (in consultation with IHS, ITs, and TOs), and make recommendations to improve the use of health care services provided under the CHS program,	9/23/2011

Section of the IHCIA Reauthorization and Extension Act of 2009 as enacted by ACA Section 10221	Title	Description	Start or Effective Date or Deadline
		including analyses of amounts reimbursed to providers, suppliers, and entities under CHS, compared to reimbursements through other public and private programs; barriers to access to health care under CHS; and adequacy of federal funding of CHS; and other matters that GAO determines appropriate.	
Section 201	Director of HIV/AIDS Prevention and Treatment	Requires the Director of the IHS office of HIV/AIDS Prevention and Treatment to submit a report to Congress describing the office's activities and findings related to HIV/AIDS prevention and treatment activities specific to Indians.	3/23/2012

Source: Prepared by the Congressional Research Service based on a review of the Patient Protection and Affordable Care Act (ACA, P.L. 111-148).

[a] Section 801 requires the President to submit a report to Congress at the time that the budget is submitted. Per 31 U.S.C. Section 1105(a) the President is required to submit his budget to Congress by the first Monday in February of the preceding fiscal year.

[b] The FY2011 budget was submitted prior to the ACA's enactment.

146 Elayne J. Heisler

Effective dates stated in terms of days, months, or years after enactment have been converted to calendar dates (e.g., 180 days is 9/19/2010; six months is 9/23/2010, etc.). Table entries for specific implementation requirements or deadlines that are not tied to a specific calendar date are presented at the end of each title. Each table entry includes the IHCIA Reauthorization and Extension Act section number as enacted by Section 10221 of the ACA; a descriptive title for each activity or requirement; a brief description of the activity or requirement; the associated start date, or effective date.[60] All of IHCIA Title VII is amended by Section 181 of the IHCIA Reauthorization and Extension Act; therefore, for requirements contained in Section 181, the subsection of IHCIA Title VII it amends is noted in parentheses.

For additional information on provisions that appear in the timeline, refer to the more detailed section summaries in the report. For definitions of acronyms used in the timeline, refer to **Appendix B**. Unless otherwise stated, references in the table to "the Secretary" refer to the Secretary of Health and Human Services (HHS).

APPENDIX B. ACRONYMS USED IN THE REPORT

ACA	Patient Protection and Affordable Care Act
AG	Attorney General
BIA	Bureau of Indian Affairs
BIE	Bureau of Indian Education
CDC	Centers for Disease Control and Prevention
CHAP	Community Health Aide Program
CHEF	Catastrophic Health Emergency Fund
CHIP	Children's Health Insurance Program
CHS	Contract Health Services
CHSDA	Contract Health Services Delivery Area
CMS	Centers for Medicare and Medicaid Services
DOD	Department of Defense
FAD	Fetal Alcohol Disorder
FAS	Fetal Alcohol Spectrum
GAO	Government Accountability Office
HCERA	Health Care and Education Reconciliation Act
HHS	Department of Health and Human Services
HIPAA	Health Insurance Portability and Accountability Act

HIT	Health Information Technology
HUD	Department of Housing and Urban Development
IHCIA	Indian Health Care Improvement Act
IHCIF	Indian Health Care Improvement Fund
IHP	Indian Health Program
IHS	Indian Health Service
IRC	Internal Revenue Code
ISDEAA	Indian Self-Determination and Education Assistance Act
IT	Indian tribe
NHHCA	Native Hawaiian Health Care Act
NHSC	National Health Service Corp
PHS	Public Health Service
PHSA	Public Health Service Act
SSA	Social Security Act
SAMSHA	Substance Abuse and Mental Health Services Administration
THP	Tribal Health Program
TO	Tribal organization
UIHP	urban Indian health project
UIO	urban Indian organization
USC	U.S. Code
VA	Department of Veterans Affairs

End Notes

[1] The ACA was subsequently amended by the Health Care and Education Reconciliation Act (HCERA, P.L. 111-152) and has since been amended by other laws. In this report, the ACA refers to the ACA as amended.

[2] CRS Report R41664, *ACA: A Brief Overview of the Law, Implementation, and Legal Challenges*, coordinated by C. Stephen Redhead. On June 28, 2011, the Supreme Court ruled, in National Federation of Independent Business v. Sebelius (NFIB), on the constitutionality of both the ACA-implemented individual mandate, which requires most U.S. residents (beginning in 2014) to carry health insurance or pay a penalty, and the ACA Medicaid expansion. The Court upheld the individual mandate as a constitutional exercise of Congress's authority to levy taxes. The penalty is to be paid by taxpayers when they file their tax returns and enforced by the Internal Revenue Service. In a separate opinion, the Court found that compelling states to participate in the ACA Medicaid expansion—which the Court determined to be essentially a new program—or risk losing their existing federal Medicaid matching funds was coercive and unconstitutional under the Spending Clause of the Constitution and the Tenth Amendment. The Court's remedy for this constitutional

148   Elayne J. Heisler

violation was to prohibit HHS from penalizing states that choose not to participate in the expansion by withholding any federal matching funds for their existing Medicaid program. However, if a state accepts the new ACA expansion funds (initially a 100% federal match), it must abide by all the expansion coverage rules. Under NFIB, all other provisions of ACA—including the Indian Health Care Improvement Act—remain fully intact and operative.

[3] P.L. 94-437, act of September 30, 1976, 90 Stat. 1400, as amended; 25 U.S.C. §1601 et seq., and 42 U.S.C. §1395qq, 1396j (and amending other sections). CRS Report R41664, *ACA: A Brief Overview of the Law, Implementation, and Legal Challenges*, coordinated by C. Stephen Redhead.

[4] As reported by the Senate Committee on Indian Affairs on December 16, 2009.

[5] See "Section 102. Findings" below.

[6] P.L. 102-573, act of October 29, 1992, 106 Stat. 4526. Previous reauthorizations occurred in 1980 (P.L. 96-537) and 1988 (P.L. 100-713), and substantial amendments were made in 1990 (P.L. 101-630, Title V).

[7] Omnibus Indian Advancement Act, P.L. 106-568, §815, act of December 27, 2000, 114 Stat. 2868, 2918.

[8] For more detailed overview information on the Indian Health Service (IHS), see CRS Report R43330, *The Indian Health Service (IHS): An Overview*, by Elayne J. Heisler.

[9] U.S. Department of Health and Human Services, Indian Health Service, IHS Fact Sheet: IHS Year 2013 Profile http://www.ihs.gov/newsroom/factsheets/ihsyear2013profile/.

[10] IHS provides services to American Indians and Alaska Natives residing in 35 states. Area offices may serve tribes in one state, such as the Alaska Area office that administers services in Alaska, or in multiple states, such as the Nashville area office that administers services for tribes on the east coast, in Alabama, Louisiana, and parts of Texas.

[11] Authorized by P.L. 93-638, the Indian Self-Determination and Education Assistance Act of January 4, 1975, 88 Stat. 2203, as amended; 25 U.S.C. 450 et seq.

[12] See "Section 102. Findings" below.

[13] Although the ACA has amended by subsequent laws, Section 10221 has not been further amended.

[14] Sec. 201(a), P.L. 81-152, act of June 30, 1949, 63 Stat. 377, 383, as amended; 40 U.S.C. 501.

[15] This program receives appropriations through the federal health center program. For more information, see http://bphc.hrsa.gov/about/specialpopulations/index.html.

[16] P.L. 92-203, act of December 18, 1971, 85 Stat. 688, as amended; 43 U.S.C. 1601 et seq.

[17] P.L. 93-638 as amended.

[18] Title V of the ACA (Health Care Workforce) authorizes a number of new programs to augment the health care workforce and amends a number of existing programs. In a number of cases ITs, TOs, and UIOs may be eligible for these programs. See CRS Report R41278, *Public Health, Workforce, Quality, and Related Provisions in ACA: Summary and Timeline*, coordinated by C. Stephen Redhead and Elayne J. Heisler.

[19] U.S. Department of Health and Human Services, Indian Health Service, "IHS Fact Sheets: Workforce," January 2010, http://www.ihs.gov/PublicAffairs/IHSBrochure/Workforce.asp.

[20] U.S. Department of Health and Human Services, Indian Health Service, *Indian Health Service: Fiscal Year 2012 Justification of Estimates for Appropriations Committees* (Rockville, MD: HHS, 2012), http://www.ihs.gov/ NonMedicalPrograms/BudgetFormulation/documents /FY%202012%20Budget%20Justification.pdf; hereinafter, IHS FY2012 Budget Justification.

[21] The text below reflects the amendments that ACA Sec. 10221(b)(1) made to this section.

The Indian Health Care Improvement Act Reauthorization ... 149

[22] P.L. 67-85, 42 Stat. 208, as amended; 25 U.S.C. §13.

[23] Beginning with the FY2014 IHS Budget Justification, the contract health service is now referred to as purchased/referred care. See U.S. Dept. of Health and Human Services, Indian Health Service, *Fiscal Year 2014 Indian Health Service Justification of Estimates*, http://www.ihs.gov/BudgetFormulation/documents/ FY2014BudgetJustification.pdf.

[24] 28 U.S.C. § 2415.

[25] P.L. 104-191, act of August 21, 1996, 110 Stat. 1936, as amended.

[26] The text below reflects the amendments that ACA Sec. 10221(b)(2) made to this section.

[27] P.L. 93-638, act of January 4, 1975, 88 Stat. 2203, as amended; 25 U.S.C. §450 et seq.

[28] 25 U.S.C. § 47

[29] GAO has released two reports on the Contract Health Service (CHS) program: (1) GAO-11-767, "Indian Health Service: Increased Oversight Needed to Ensure Accuracy of Data Used for Estimating Contract Health Service Need." See http://www.gao.gov/new.items /d11767.pdf, September 23, 2011; and (2) GAO-12-446, "Indian Health Service: Action Needed to Ensure Equitable Allocation of Resources for the Contract Health Service Program." See http://www.gao.gov/assets/600/591631.pdf, June 15, 2012.

[30] IHS FY2012 Budget Justification.

[31] The four types of facilities are inpatient health care facilities, outpatient health care facilities, staff quarters, and youth regional treatment centers.

[32] The specified workgroup and advisory board existed prior to enactment.

[33] IHCIA Section 801, which was not amended by the ACA, requires the President, each fiscal year to submit a number of required reports to Congress describing various IHCIA-authorized programs and other topics related to Indian health.

[34] U.S. Dept. of Health and Human Services, Indian Health Service, *Fiscal Year 2014 Indian Health Service Justification of Estimates*, http://www.ihs.gov/BudgetFormulation /documents/FY2014BudgetJustification.pdf.

[35] In order to be eligible for the CHS program, American Indians and Alaska Natives must be eligible for IHS services and live within a specified geographic area called a contract health service delivery area, or CHSDA.

[36] Section 508 of American Recovery and Reinvestment Act (P.L. 111-5) exempted American Indians and Alaska Natives from premiums and cost-sharing in Medicaid and CHIP. Sec. 2901 of the ACA also includes provisions to facilitate enrollment in Medicaid and CHIP. See description in CRS Report R41210, *Medicaid and the State Children's Health Insurance Program (CHIP) Provisions in ACA: Summary and Timeline*, by Evelyne P. Baumrucker et al.

[37] A memorandum of understanding between IHS and the VA was signed on October 1, 2010; see http://www.ihs.gov/ announcements/documents/3-OD-11-0006.pdf.

[38] For information on VA reimbursement, see U.S. Department of Veteran's Affairs, "VA and Indian Health Service Announce National Reimbursement Agreement," press release, December 6, 2012.

[39] Under 5 U.S.C. Chapter 89.

[40] Under 5 U.S.C. Chapter 87.

[41] The Navajo reservation is located in parts of Arizona, Utah, and New Mexico.

[42] See U.S. Department of Health and Human Services, Indian Health Service, "Urban Indian Health Program: Program Overview." At http://www.ihs.gov/NonMedicalPrograms/Urban /Overview.asp.

[43] IHS FY2012 Budget Justification.

150   Elayne J. Heisler

[44] IHS is forbidden to bill or charge Indians (see 25 U.S.C. 1681 and 25 USC 458aaa-14), but IHCIA Title V does not prohibit UIHPs from charging their patients. "Section 197. Tribal Health Program Option for Cost Sharing" described below permits some THPs to charge for services.

[45] U.S. Dept. of Health and Human Services, Indian Health Service, *Fiscal Year 2014 Indian Health Service Justification of Estimates*, http://www.ihs.gov/BudgetFormulation /documents/FY2014BudgetJustification.pdf.

[46] JCAHO now goes by the title The Joint Commission (TJC).

[47] HHS and the Department of Interior amended a 2009 memorandum of agreement to incorporate the requirements of the new IHCIA provision. See http://www.ihs.gov /publicinfo/publications/ihsmanual/part3/pt3chapt18/moua.htm.

[48] See Title IV of P.L. 99-570.

[49] These locations are the Tanana Chiefs Conference, Incorporated and the Southeast Alaska Regional Health Corporation.

[50] The BIA's educational programs were transferred to a new agency, the Bureau of Indian Education (BIE), in 2006.

[51] P.L. 101-630, Title IV, act of November 28, 1990, 104 Stat. 4544, as amended; 25 U.S.C. § 3202 et seq., 18 U.S.C. §1169.

[52] No funds have been appropriated to support this program.

[53] 5 U.S.C. § 552.

[54] For more information about the National Health Service Corps, see U.S. Department of Health and Human Services, Health Resources and Services Administration, "National Health Service Corps," http://nhsc.hrsa.gov/.

[55] In October 2011, the Department of Justice released "Indian Health Care Improvement Act, Report Required by 25 U.S.C. 1680q(b)(2)." See http://www.justice.gov/tribal/docs/ihia-pdmp-rpt-to-congress.pdf.

[56] GAO has released three reports on the CHS program: (1) GAO-11-767, "Indian Health Service: Increased Oversight Needed to Ensure Accuracy of Data Used for Estimating Contract Health Service Need." http://www.gao.gov/ new.items/d11767.pdf, September 23, 2011; (2) GAO-12-446, "Indian Health Service: Action Needed to Ensure Equitable Allocation of Resources for the Contract Health Service Program," http://www.gao.gov/assets/600/ 591631.pdf, June 15, 2012; and (3) U.S. Government Accountability Office, *Indian Health Service: Capping Payments for Nonhospital Services Could Save Millions of Dollars for Contract Health Services*, 13-272, April 11, 2013, http://www.gao.gov/products/GAO-13-272.

[57] P.L. 101-381 as amended.

[58] Prior to the mark-up of the IHCIA Reauthorization and Extension Act by the Committee on Indian Affairs, the Act included provisions to amend the SSA. These provisions were either struck during the mark-up or were struck by Sec. 10221(b)(4).

[59] This program receives appropriations through the federal health center program. For more information, see http://bphc.hrsa.gov/about/specialpopulations.htm and Appendix A of CRS Report R42433, *Federal Health Centers*, by Elayne J. Heisler.

[60] This report does not track actions taken in response to the deadline or effective date; however, this information is available to congressional clients from the author.

INDEX

A

abuse, 15, 82, 121, 135
access, 11, 16, 22, 60, 62, 67, 71, 75, 81, 82, 84, 94, 106, 118, 120, 122, 124, 125, 131, 132, 136, 145
accounting, 19, 79
accreditation, 18, 125
administrative efficiency, 19
administrative support, 125
adolescent behavior, 107
adolescents, 83, 127
adults, 47, 124
Affordable Care Act, i, iii, v, vii, ix, x, 21, 22, 36, 39, 40, 69, 70, 88, 89, 91, 93, 94, 145, 146
age, 15
agencies, 4, 13, 23, 24, 25, 52, 78, 81, 107, 114, 122, 125, 130, 135, 136, 138, 144
AIDS, 137, 145
Alaska village clinics, vii, 2, 8, 9, 10
alcoholism, 72, 130
American Recovery and Reinvestment Act, 149
appropriations, viii, ix, 2, 19, 20, 21, 23, 32, 42, 61, 65, 70, 72, 73, 74, 75, 78, 79, 82, 83, 84, 89, 90, 95, 96, 97, 98, 101, 102, 108, 115, 116, 129, 131, 138, 148, 150
Appropriations Committee, 90, 148
assault, 129

assessment, 78, 125, 135
assets, 32, 33, 90, 149, 150
Attorney General, 130, 146
audit, 41, 79, 116
authority(s), vii, x, 1, 2, 3, 4, 7, 11, 13, 17, 21, 33, 40, 70, 72, 73, 80, 87, 88, 95, 97, 99, 106, 113, 121, 138, 147
authorized programs, 21, 95, 149
awareness, 135

B

barriers, 62, 136, 145
base, 101, 127
behavioral problems, 124
behaviors, 16, 24
beneficiaries, viii, 2, 3, 4, 9, 11, 13, 14, 15, 16, 22, 24, 57, 61, 63, 64, 87, 117, 118
benefits, 3, 17, 55, 62, 63, 74, 84, 85, 89, 91, 98, 115, 117, 119, 120
BIA, 20, 21, 22, 25, 26, 27, 28, 36, 125, 128, 146, 150
BIE, 146
blindness, 34
blood, 15
bonuses, 18
building code, 18
Bureau of Indian Affairs (BIA), 5, 25, 26, 27, 32, 36, 86, 91, 105, 146

152 Index

Bureau of Indian Education (BIE), 132, 146, 150
burn, 14

C

cancer, 73, 97, 101, 106
cancer screening, 73, 97, 106
car accidents, 57
CDC, 106, 107, 146
Census, 4, 6, 24, 25, 26, 27, 28, 32, 36
certification, 99, 108, 125, 129
CFR, 33
challenges, viii, 37, 40, 60, 62, 65
child abuse, 81, 127
childcare, 126
childhood, 129
children, 9, 25, 80, 83, 120, 124, 127, 130, 134
CHIP, ix, x, 12, 18, 23, 24, 34, 69, 70, 71, 76, 79, 83, 87, 89, 90, 115, 116, 117, 136, 144, 146, 149
cholesterol, 15
CHS payments, viii, 37, 40, 58, 83
CHS program, viii, 37, 38, 39, 40, 41, 42, 43, 44, 45, 47, 48, 49, 50, 51, 52, 53, 54, 55, 56, 57, 58, 59, 60, 61, 62, 63, 64, 65, 66, 67, 73, 83, 90, 97, 110, 140, 144, 149, 150
CHS providers, viii, 37, 38, 40, 52, 77, 83
City, 8, 65, 121
civil action, 104
Clean Water Act, 89
clients, 150
closure, 111
collaboration, 15, 19, 74, 98, 124, 131
colleges, 82, 107
community(s), vii, 1, 5, 6, 12, 16, 20, 27, 36, 65, 73, 76, 77, 79, 82, 85, 86, 96, 97, 99, 100, 103, 105, 106, 109, 113, 114, 125, 126, 127, 128, 129, 131, 135, 144
community-based services, 77, 103
compensation, 66, 104
complexity, 39, 57
compliance, 55, 79

complications, 15, 16, 102
conference, 109, 121
congress, 2, 5, 9, 20, 21, 22, 31, 35, 36, 69, 72, 78, 82, 88, 89, 100, 101, 107, 108, 110, 111, 115, 120, 123, 129, 131, 133, 136, 137, 138, 139, 140, 141, 142, 144, 145, 147, 149, 150
consent, 102, 123
conservation, 90
Constitution, 2, 88, 147
construction, viii, 2, 16, 17, 18, 20, 72, 73, 78, 89, 97, 110, 111, 112, 113, 114, 121, 140
consulting, 116
consumer price index, 135, 143
cooperation, 125, 127, 128
cooperative agreements, 112
coordination, 80, 82, 83, 115, 121, 125, 129, 130, 135, 136, 144
cosmetic, 44
cost, 14, 17, 48, 67, 79, 84, 85, 87, 94, 102, 117, 125, 135, 141, 143, 149
counseling, 11, 12, 82, 126
course work, 126
covering, 83
criminal violence, 66
CSCs, 19
curricula, 82, 129
curriculum, 83, 132

D

damages, 104
data collection, 131
data set, 106
deaths, 35
deficiencies, 77, 101, 116, 139
denial, 61
dental, viii, 2, 6, 9, 10, 11, 12, 43, 71, 77, 99, 100
dental care, 9, 10
dentist, 99
Department of Defense, 74, 80, 98, 115, 146

Index

Department of Health and Human Services, vii, ix, 1, 2, 27, 32, 33, 34, 35, 36, 39, 70, 71, 88, 89, 90, 91, 95, 146, 148, 149, 150
Department of Justice, 150
Department of the Interior, 20, 25, 82, 142
detention, 131
detoxification, 127
diabetes, viii, 2, 3, 15, 34, 72, 73, 77, 95, 97, 101, 102
dialysis, 102
direct payment, 116
disability, 120
disaster, 102
disbursement, 110
disclosure, 133
disease rate, 17
diseases, viii, 2, 16, 17, 20, 72, 77, 81, 107, 121, 134, 139
disorder, 15, 82, 128
distribution, 78, 110, 134
domestic violence, 129
draft, 64
drinking water, 17
drug abuse, 81, 127, 135

E

education, 11, 16, 58, 76, 81, 82, 99, 105, 107, 108, 120, 125, 126, 128, 129, 131
educational materials, 131
educational programs, 84, 99, 138, 150
elders, 125
eligibility criteria, 13, 14, 45, 103
emergency, viii, 2, 9, 10, 11, 13, 14, 16, 38, 43, 44, 45, 57, 71, 79, 99, 106, 127, 134
employees, 73, 74, 76, 80, 97, 98, 100, 103, 113, 119, 128
employers, 84, 89
employment, 20, 42, 122, 123, 126
end-stage renal disease, 66
enrollment, ix, 25, 26, 27, 36, 48, 62, 70, 76, 79, 80, 84, 85, 91, 115, 116, 117, 118, 149
epidemiology, 77, 106
equipment, 18, 78, 102, 113, 114, 122

ethnic groups, 15
evidence, 35, 41
examinations, 129
exercise, viii, 2, 4, 23, 88, 147
expertise, 131

F

FAD, 128, 146
families, 66, 94, 124
family members, 127, 131
family therapy, 126
family violence, 127, 130
FAS, 82, 109, 124, 146
federal agency, vii, 1, 2, 19, 100, 113, 127
federal funds, 83
federal government, viii, 2, 4, 5, 19, 28, 31, 48, 62, 66, 67, 79, 86, 90, 91, 122
federal law, 83, 100, 137
Federal Register, 91, 125
federal reservations, vii, 1, 6
fetal alcohol syndrome, 82, 109, 124
financial, 19, 84, 117, 124
fiscal year 2009, 52
flexibility, 60
formula, 90, 110

G

gastroenteritis, 20
General Accounting Office (GAO), viii, 34, 35, 37, 38, 40, 44, 46, 49, 50, 51, 57, 66, 67, 90, 110, 112, 136, 140, 141, 144, 145, 146, 149, 150
General Services Administration, 122
goods and services, 81
governance, 7, 18, 19, 22, 23, 65, 71, 83, 88, 95
governments, 21
GPRA, 39, 52, 53, 54, 64, 67
grant programs, ix, 14, 70, 132
grants, vii, 1, 3, 9, 11, 15, 33, 65, 71, 73, 74, 75, 78, 79, 80, 81, 82, 95, 97, 98, 106,

154 Index

107, 112, 114, 115, 117, 120, 121, 122, 125, 126, 128, 129, 130, 131, 132, 139
growth, 94
guidance, 42, 54, 123
guidelines, 118, 127

H

Hawaii, 7, 10, 84
Health and Human Services, 10, 23, 32, 65, 74, 89, 146, 149, 150
health care costs, 15
health care coverage, viii, 37, 39, 40, 47, 48, 61, 62, 63, 80
health care professionals, 18, 107
health care programs, 11, 80, 101, 119, 120, 124
health centers, vii, 2, 8, 9, 10, 18, 35, 72, 78, 99, 110, 112
health condition, viii, x, 2, 4, 14, 21, 72, 93, 95
health education, viii, 2, 3, 9, 11, 12, 16, 77, 83, 96, 101, 137
health information, 81, 106, 120
health insurance, ix, 47, 66, 69, 71, 73, 84, 85, 86, 88, 89, 91, 94, 104, 117, 147
health practitioners, 77, 99, 113
health problems, 127, 128, 130
health programs, vii, 1, 3, 7, 13, 15, 77, 81, 88, 90, 101, 124, 127
health promotion, 15, 16, 76, 77, 81, 83, 96, 99, 109, 120, 136, 137, 138
health stations, vii, 2, 8, 79, 112, 141
health status, ix, 3, 61, 69, 72, 95, 101, 108, 110, 139
hepatitis, 16, 17, 72, 107
HHS, vii, ix, 1, 2, 6, 19, 20, 23, 33, 35, 39, 64, 70, 71, 74, 80, 81, 84, 86, 88, 90, 95, 96, 98, 105, 114, 122, 129, 137, 146, 148, 150
history, 4, 32
HIV, ix, 70, 74, 83, 98, 137, 145
HIV/AIDS, ix, 70, 74, 83, 98, 137, 145
homes, 17, 20
homicide, 130

hospice, 77, 103
hospitalization, 16
hospitals, vii, 1, 8, 12, 18, 22, 40, 72, 76, 78, 110, 112
House, 23, 31
House of Representatives, 31
household income, 67
housing, 129
Housing and Urban Development (HUD), 147
HPV, 17
human, 17, 124

I

identification, 24, 26, 36, 105
immunization, 16, 17
improvements, 63, 116, 130
incidence, x, 72, 93, 95, 102, 130
income, 48, 66, 67, 84, 85, 90, 91
increased access, 63
increased workload, 59, 65
Indian Health Care Improvement Act, v, vii, viii, ix, x, 1, 2, 3, 5, 19, 21, 31, 33, 34, 36, 69, 70, 72, 85, 88, 91, 93, 94, 147, 148, 150
Indian Health Service, i, iii, v, vii, ix, x, 1, 2, 7, 10, 24, 26, 27, 32, 33, 34, 35, 36, 37, 38, 39, 66, 67, 69, 71, 74, 88, 89, 90, 91, 93, 94, 147, 148, 149, 150
Indian reservation, 24, 71, 95
Indian Tribes, vii, ix, 1, 3, 7, 10, 28, 67, 70, 84
individuals, 5, 6, 15, 17, 24, 25, 34, 42, 47, 62, 66, 67, 76, 83, 84, 85, 86, 94, 108, 134
industry, 53
infant mortality, 20, 72
inflation, 74, 83, 98, 135
infrastructure, 81, 122, 131
injury(s), 83, 136, 144
injury prevention, 83, 136, 144
institutions, 130
insurance coverage, ix, 22, 70, 71, 84, 85, 91
integration, 112

Index

interagency coordination, 137
internal consistency, 41
Internal Revenue Service, 88, 147
Intervals, 49, 52
intervention, 126, 129, 130, 131, 132
intervention strategies, 132
investment, 17
IRC, 84, 85, 147
issues, 15, 23, 38, 44, 45, 47, 55, 59, 63, 67, 128

J

jurisdiction, viii, 2, 4, 5, 23, 86
justification, 74, 89, 111, 112, 143

K

kidney, 15

L

labor force, 27
law enforcement, 130, 135
laws, viii, 2, 19, 101, 104, 147, 148
lead, vii, 1, 2, 19, 39
leadership, 123
legislation, viii, 2, 3, 4, 19, 23, 28
litigation, 104
local community, 15, 127
local government, 104, 134, 136, 144
Louisiana, 6, 88, 148

M

majority, viii, 2, 12, 28, 38, 48, 58, 127
mammography, 105
management, 16, 19, 21, 74, 81, 98, 120
marital status, 91
marriage, 126
materials, 105

medical, viii, 2, 3, 11, 14, 34, 43, 54, 56, 61, 62, 63, 65, 66, 71, 77, 83, 91, 99, 102, 104, 118, 129, 131, 133
medical benefit package, viii, 2, 12, 71
medical care, 11, 91
Medicare, ix, x, 12, 14, 18, 21, 22, 23, 24, 32, 34, 43, 55, 66, 67, 69, 70, 71, 72, 74, 76, 79, 80, 81, 83, 87, 88, 89, 91, 94, 95, 98, 103, 115, 116, 117, 120, 134, 136, 144, 146
Medicare Modernization Act, 34
medicine, 76
membership, 4, 5, 24, 25, 26, 32, 86, 100
membership criteria, 5, 32
mental health, ix, 9, 15, 70, 72, 75, 77, 82, 124, 125, 126, 127, 128, 130, 131, 132, 141
mental illness, 105, 127, 142
methamphetamine treatment, viii, 2
methodology, 78, 111
Mexico, 8, 82, 90, 149
mission, viii, 2
models, 126, 128, 129, 130
modifications, 110
mortality, 20

N

National Health Service, 19, 134, 147, 150
national policy, ix, x, 21, 69, 72, 93, 95
Native Americans, 33, 66
Navajo Nation, 80, 120, 141
negotiating, 21, 118
neurodevelopmental disorders, 124
neutral, 100
North America, 36
nurses, 16, 18, 76, 99
nursing, viii, 2, 11, 16, 44, 71, 76, 103
nursing care, 16

O

obstacles, 130, 142

156 Index

officials, viii, 37, 38, 39, 41, 46, 53, 54, 55, 56, 57, 58, 59, 60, 61, 65, 135
Oklahoma, vii, 1, 6, 8, 41, 65, 121
on behavioral health concerns, vii, 2, 8
opportunities, 74, 75, 98, 137
organ, 6, 44
outpatient, vii, viii, 1, 2, 8, 9, 10, 12, 14, 78, 127, 149
outreach, 11, 62, 80, 132
overlap, 3
oversight, 24, 40
ownership, 5, 86

P

parents, 25
parity, 101
participants, 14, 116
Pascua Yaqui Tribe of Arizona, 32
patient care, 8
penalties, 84, 85, 87
per capita income, 90
permit, ix, 21, 70, 81, 87, 95, 100, 112, 121, 122, 138
personal communication, 27, 32
physical therapy, 59
physicians, 18, 20, 40, 76, 99
pneumonia, 17, 35
policy, 3, 19, 21, 96, 108, 123
policy issues, 96
population, x, 3, 4, 6, 8, 12, 15, 17, 21, 24, 25, 27, 28, 32, 33, 36, 62, 72, 74, 75, 79, 83, 93, 95, 98, 108, 109, 113, 120, 132, 135, 143
population growth, 25
potential benefits, 114
poverty, 47, 67, 84, 87
PPACA, viii, 37, 39, 40, 41, 47, 61, 62, 63, 64, 66, 67, 89, 91
PRC, 13, 14, 15, 34
pregnancy, 5, 86
premature death, x, 93, 95
prescription drug abuse, 135, 144
prescription drugs, 74, 87, 98, 133

President, ix, x, 21, 69, 70, 93, 94, 111, 123, 135, 140, 143, 145, 149
President Obama, ix, x, 69, 70, 93, 94
prevention, viii, ix, 2, 15, 16, 17, 70, 74, 75, 76, 77, 81, 82, 84, 96, 98, 99, 101, 105, 106, 107, 109, 121, 124, 125, 126, 127, 128, 129, 130, 131, 132, 134, 135, 136, 137, 139, 142, 145
preventive care, viii, 2, 3, 9, 12, 61
preventive screenings, viii, 2, 12
private education, 138
private sector, 18
professionals, 9, 18, 76, 99, 100, 107, 109, 119
program staff, 59, 60, 63, 64, 65
project, 21, 79, 111, 112, 114, 128, 130, 131, 141, 147
protection, 87, 125
psychiatry, 82, 130, 132
psychologist, 126
psychology, 82, 107, 126, 130, 132
psychotherapy, 15, 131
public health, viii, 2, 11, 16, 23, 71, 88, 89, 106
Public Health Service Act, 9, 120, 147

Q

qualifications, 105
quality assurance, 83, 133

R

race, 4, 24, 25, 26, 27, 28
rape, 129
recognition, 5, 86, 90, 132, 134
recognized tribe, vii, 1, 3, 5, 7, 25, 36, 40, 42, 57, 67, 80, 86, 87, 96, 120, 134
recommendations, 38, 64, 101, 130, 136, 144
recovery, 104
recruiting, 18, 99
reform(s), ix, x, 69, 70, 88, 93, 94
registries, 102

Index

157

regulations, 41, 42, 56, 83, 102, 107, 110, 113, 114, 133
rehabilitation, 44, 124, 125, 127, 129
reimburse, 14, 19, 134
reliability, 41
renal replacement therapy, 44
rent, 113
repair, 113
resources, 3, 13, 16, 42, 45, 54, 56, 57, 59, 60, 61, 66, 75, 101, 108, 121, 124, 125
response, 52, 65, 138, 150
restrictions, 83
rights, 104, 119
risk, 14, 88, 102, 131, 147
risk factors, 131
rules, 14, 48, 57, 58, 60, 61, 88, 148
rural areas, 18, 99

S

safety, 106
SAMHSA, 82, 130, 131, 132
scholarship, 18, 19, 76, 84, 96, 107, 137
school, 9, 77, 83, 84, 99, 101, 128, 132, 135
scope, 125
secondary education, 126
self-destructive behavior, 105, 127, 142
Senate, 23, 35, 66, 73, 123, 148
service provider, 122
sewage, 17, 72, 78, 111
sexual abuse, 82, 129
sexual violence, 82, 129, 142
shortage, 19
showing, 53, 59
signs, 17
small businesses, 47
smallpox, 28
Social Security, ix, 69, 115, 147
social services, 15, 124
socioeconomic status, 132
solid waste, 17, 72, 78, 111
South Dakota, 89, 133
specialists, 12
spending, 94

SSA, ix, 69, 70, 71, 73, 76, 79, 87, 89, 105, 106, 115, 117, 118, 119, 147, 150
stabilization, 134
staffing, 38, 39, 55, 59, 64, 102
State Children's Health Insurance Program, ix, 12, 23, 69, 71, 74, 89, 90, 97, 115, 149
statute of limitations, 104
statutes, viii, 2, 37, 41
structure, 23, 75, 108, 127
substance abuse, vii, x, 2, 8, 9, 15, 21, 72, 82, 94, 95, 109, 124, 125, 128
Substance Abuse and Mental Health Services Administration (SAMHSA), 75, 89, 129, 131
substitutes, 91
suicide, viii, 2, 15, 72, 74, 75, 82, 95, 98, 124, 127, 130, 131, 132, 143
suicide rate, 131
supervision, 99, 103
suppliers, 136, 145
support services, 129
Supreme Court, 19, 35, 88, 147
surplus, 81, 122
surveillance, 15, 16, 17

T

Tanana Chiefs Conference, 150
target, viii, 2, 14, 38, 52, 54, 55
Task Force, 31
tax credits, 48
taxes, 88, 147
taxpayers, 88, 147
technical assistance, 12, 17, 42, 72, 78, 105, 106, 107, 108, 111, 113, 124, 137
technician, 126
techniques, 130
technology(s), 12, 24, 81, 82, 120
telecommunications, 117
teleconferencing, 99
therapist, 77, 99, 100, 126
therapy, 99
Title I, 36, 73, 74, 76, 77, 78, 79, 81, 87, 96, 97, 99, 101, 110, 115, 120, 137, 150

Index

Title II, 36, 73, 77, 78, 79, 87, 96, 97, 101, 110, 137
Title IV, 74, 79, 97, 115, 120, 150
Title V, vii, 1, 3, 15, 22, 33, 35, 74, 80, 81, 82, 83, 90, 98, 119, 120, 121, 122, 124, 129, 133, 135, 146, 148, 150
tracks, 53
training, 12, 18, 19, 58, 76, 82, 99, 105, 125, 126, 128, 129, 131, 132, 135
training programs, 130
translation, 15
transport, 106
transportation, 17, 73, 97, 106, 117
trauma, 44
treaties, 2, 28, 62
treatment, vii, viii, ix, x, 2, 8, 9, 15, 21, 22, 70, 72, 74, 75, 81, 82, 94, 98, 102, 105, 107, 118, 121, 124, 125, 126, 127, 129, 130, 131, 137, 142, 145, 149
Tribal Organizations, vii, 1, 3
tuberculosis, 35, 77
turnover, 58

U

U.S. Department of Commerce, 27, 32, 36
U.S. Department of the Interior, 27, 32, 36, 91
UIOs, vii, ix, 1, 3, 5, 8, 11, 15, 21, 25, 33, 70, 71, 72, 74, 75, 80, 81, 86, 87, 95, 98, 99, 104, 106, 109, 112, 117, 120, 121, 122, 124, 125, 126, 129, 130, 131, 135, 137, 148
uniform, 24
United, v, 5, 31, 37, 65, 75, 83, 85, 103, 104, 107, 109, 110, 119, 131, 136

United States, v, 5, 31, 37, 65, 75, 83, 85, 103, 104, 107, 109, 110, 119, 131, 136
universities, 107
urban, ix, 3, 11, 21, 25, 28, 32, 33, 69, 71, 72, 74, 80, 81, 95, 98, 108, 109, 120, 121, 127, 130, 147
urban areas, 3, 28, 71, 95, 120, 127, 130
Urban Indian Organizations, vii, 1, 3, 25, 121

V

vacancies, 18, 35, 77, 89, 100
variations, 55
victims, 14, 66, 102, 129, 142
vision, 34

W

wage rate, 78, 89
Washington, 27, 31, 32, 35, 36, 66, 67
waste, 17
waste disposal, 17
water, 16, 17, 72, 78, 111
water supplies, 16
workers, 73, 97, 99, 104, 131
workforce, viii, x, 2, 4, 17, 19, 65, 73, 76, 82, 88, 89, 93, 95, 97, 99, 148
working hours, 112

Y

youth regional treatment centers, vii, 2, 8, 149